THE
ANTI-AGING
WEIGHT LOSS
PROGRAM

Also by Dr. Hans Kugler

Dr. Kugler's Seven Keys to a Longer Life

THE ANTI-AGING WEIGHT LOSS PROGRAM

DR. HANS J. KUGLER

When you're slim and youthful, the
whole world smiles at you.

STEIN AND DAY/Publishers/New York

First published in 1985
Copyright © 1985 by Hans J. Kugler, Ph.D.
All rights reserved, Stein and Day, Incorporated
Designed by Louis A. Ditizio
Printed in the United States of America
STEIN AND DAY/*Publishers*
Scarborough House
Briarcliff Manor, NY 10510

Library of Congress Cataloging in Publication Data

Kugler, Hans J.
  The anti-aging weight-loss program.

  Bibliography: p.
  Includes index.
  1. Reducing diets.   2. Aging—Prevention.
3. Longevity.   I. Title.
RM222.2.K84   1985   613.2′5   84-40727
ISBN 0-8128-3028-8

Acknowledgments

I WOULD LIKE TO EXPRESS MY SINCERE
APPRECIATION TO:

John Drammis, M.D.
Cosmetic and Youth Surgeon, Chicago
For providing me with detailed information regarding surgi-
cal methods for body-shaping and looking younger. Dr.
Drammis is one of the leading surgeons involved in perfecting
these new and fascinating techniques.

Mr. Rudy Smith,
President of the Holiday Spa Health Clubs, California, and
his wife, Virginia, for their idealism in furthering the goals of
the health and physical fitness movement and for being such
good examples by practicing what they preach.

Ms. Francoise Nigron
El Segundo, California,
For her patience in editing the manuscript of this book, and
for suggesting the illustrations used here and in the Holistic
and Preventive UP-DATE.

The Leaders of HTC,
the Health and Tennis Corporation of America, for so effectively bringing the fitness and health message to the population at large.

The Board Members of the
International Academy of Holistic Health & Medicine
For their efforts, research, and endurance in promoting the
principles in holistic health, medicine, and aging.

Prof. Franz Schmid, M.D.   Prof. Robert Mendelsohn, M.D.
Dr. John Thie, D.C.   Garry Gordon, M.D.
Richard Passwater, Ph.D.   Harold Rosenberg, M.D.
Harvey Ross, M.D.   Bernard Rimland, Ph.D.
Morton Walker, D.P.M.   David Wong, M.D.
Susan Smith Jones, Ph.D.   John Drammis, M.D.
Charles (Chuck) Coker, MA   Sidney Dupois, Pharm.D.,
                                       Ph.D.

Contents

List of Tables

List of Figures

INTRODUCTION
What this is all about.

Not another diet book!
No, definitely not!
Why not? What makes this book so different from any other weight-loss book?

This is both a scientific approach to weight loss and one that also interferes with many of the causes of aging. If you follow the advice given in this book, you *will* shed those extra pounds. In addition, your weight loss will be safe, permanent, and *rejuvenating*. And since you have a choice over many of the factors that can be applied, doing it will be easy and fun.

There are at least nine different factors that make major contributions to any weight loss or weight gain; they range from very general factors (that apply to everybody) to highly specific ones (important only for a small percentage of the population). Evaluating these factors, and determining which ones apply to you, will make it crystal clear what *you* should be doing in respect to your overall diet, specific foods, physical activity, eating patterns, or specific supplements in order to assure *your* permanent weight loss. Applying the

11

correct factors for your specific situation and biochemical individuality is what allows it to be easy and fun. If weight loss is truly difficult and a pain, it means only one thing: You are not doing it right. I have seen dozens of people who suffer through strenuous exercises when their real weight problem is the faulty composition of their diets. Others exercise six times a week the wrong way, with little to show for it, when they could have exercised only three times a week and could have had a guaranteed weight loss. Then there are the people who put themselves under extreme distress with weird diets, not knowing that by making a mere adjustment of one or another specific biochemical factor, they could have an almost immediate weight loss.

Why do more than absolutely necessary when by *doing it the right way* you can have the key to easy weight loss.

Most weight-loss books fall into one of two classes:

1. They are written by nutritional ignoramuses. The nutrition, when evaluated relative to established standards, is very risky and can do you a lot of harm; it is often so bad that your body has no choice but to lose weight. This not only endangers your health but also induces a tremendous acceleration of the rate of aging. Even worse, if you go back to your normal eating routine, these pounds go back on much faster. This is called the yo-yo syndrome.

2. They are written by good scientists who utilize only the most basic weight-loss principles. Even though theoretically correct, this approach works only for a very small number of people, and it doesn't work at all for the rest of the population because the latest weight-loss factors are not included.

Both types of diet books are unsuccessful for their followers or far too difficult.

The proof is in the fact that despite all the weight-loss books on the market, 60 percent of the American population is overweight.

To be truly successful, and to make weight loss easy, we must evaluate *all* contributing weight-loss factors and determine which ones are to be applied to guarantee *your* weight loss. Then the *doing it*, the most important part in a weight-loss program, becomes easy.

To give you the fastest possible results, each chapter discusses a specific aspect of the weight-loss picture, and the first page often carries a short quiz that quickly evaluates whether or not you should concern yourself with the material in a particular chapter. If the quiz determines that you are already doing things right, or that this specific weight-loss factor doesn't apply to you, you can just move on to the next chapter. After all, why do more than what is necessary?

In Part 1 we discuss the nine weight-loss factors, explain the basic supporting research, and make minimum recommendations to get maximum results. After discussing each weight-loss factor, you will be asked to make a check mark in Figure 10.1 (chapter 10). By the time we have discussed all of the weight-loss factors, your personal weight-loss profile will have emerged and you will know exactly what *you* have to do to lose those pounds successfully and easily.

Most people don't recognize that having a disease-risk factor in one's life can age them as much as actually being old according to their chronological age. Supporting research was published by Professor Bernard Strehler, one of the leading gerontologists in the United States.

Many weight-loss factors—from general nutrition to specific vitamins, specific minerals, stress, and physical activity—contribute to aging and condense the entire life span so that "old age," with all its signs and symptoms, sets in earlier. Applying these factors correctly increases a life span and delays or prevents aging.

After you've read part 1, you'll know everything you have to know in order to shed *your* excess weight, safely. This leaves only two things for us to do: (1) make you aware of obstacles that could make your weight loss a failure (part 2), and (2) Make things foolproof and teach you how to *do it* and do it right (part 3).

In Part 2 we discuss a number of obstacles that could make your weight loss a failure. This ranges from drinking too many calories (not just alcoholic drinks) to eating disorders such as binging, bulimia, or food allergies that can make you crave certain foods. For each one of these problem areas, the weight-loss factors discussed in part 1 take on a different priority.

In a separate research project, we are working with people who binge or suffer from bulimia. Our success rate is higher than that of the major eating disorder clinics. If you take our advice and follow it precisely, the anti-aging weight-loss program will also help you rid yourself of these eating disorders.

Whether you like to cook, prefer prepackaged meals, or eat out all the time, here is the right advice for healthy nutrition.

In part 3 we simplify, review, give direct advice on how to prepare your own foods, and explain which shortcut weight-loss diets have failed the test. We also outline how to reward yourself for your weight-loss success and how to use our weight-loss checklist to make sure that nothing important is overlooked. We make doing it foolproof.

At this point you'll know everything you have to know about losing those extra pounds. Since the advice given in each chapter can be translated into a definite weight loss, you can now combine what you've learned to accelerate your results. You also don't have to be perfect: If the instructions in one chapter are not exactly to your liking, you can just do the absolute minimum and balance the overall program by stressing other instructions a little bit more.

Combining several modalities, from nutrition to exercise and various aspects of motivation, has been proven highly successful by a number of weight-loss researchers. On the basis of these and other studies, Dr. Jack Wilmore and his associates have worked out therapeutic guidelines for weight control that were published in the *American Journal of Clinical Nutrition* and that are also included in our approach.

Our statistics show that more than 80 percent of all people would lose weight if they followed the instructions of the first six chapters only. It's so easy, and understanding what healthy weight-loss is allows you to make choices and fit the program to your personal taste.

And that's what this book is all about: Doing it *right* and having *you* take charge of your own life.

In closing this introduction, let me emphasize again that the success of our program is based on evaluating the many weight-loss factors and in determining exactly which ones are to be applied to guarantee *your* permanent weight loss. Many times, just one single factor can be the critical point for making your weight-loss program a success or failure. It might even be the key to your weight problem. If it applies, don't ignore it. Now, get ready to *do it.*

Part 1

THE NINE
WEIGHT-LOSS
FACTORS AND THEIR
ANTI-AGING PROPERTIES

A Better Tomorrow Starts Today

Did you read the introduction?
It's important!

1

YOUR METABOLISM—FAST OR SLOW?

Biochemical individuality explains why what's good for the goose can be fattening for the gander.

> Having a slow metabolism is not always a disadvantage. According to research in the field of aging, it can also mean a slowing down of the entire aging process.
>
> Gary Gordon, M.D.
> Nutrition and weight-loss specialist

> I have exactly what I had two years ago, only it's a little bit lower.
>
> Gypsy Rose Lee

CHECK YOURSELF

Some people are slow or fast oxidizers, or we say that they have a slow or fast metabolism. Recently, research results demonstrated that the effectiveness of our metabolism is very much determined by the number of sodium-potassium pumps in our body and the amount of the body's lean muscle mass. We can use the following data to determine if you have a slow or fast metabolism.

1. Do you often feel cold; are you the first one to put on a sweater? YES NO

2. Do you have great difficulty controlling your weight by merely cutting down on your food intake? YES NO

3. Do you feel that you have a slow
   metabolism?   YES   NO

If you have answered "NO" to all three questions, you can
check "Doesn't apply" for item 1 in Figure 10.1, chapter 10,
and move on to the next chapter. If you have one or more
"YES" answers, you must read this chapter.

BIOCHEMICAL INDIVIDUALITY

The expression *biochemical individuality* was coined by the
famous Texas University professor, Roger Williams. It simply means that we are all different in respect of what is going
on in our body, that we must adjust our nutrition to our
personal life-style, and that achieving the best possible state
of health and preventing aging must be a very personal and
individual approach.

Depending on activity, age, sex, stress situation, environ-
mental factors, and some of the factors that we will discuss in
the following chapters—which determine our personal metabolism—each one of us has a very specific daily caloric
maintenance level (DCML), also referred to as the daily
caloric need to maintain a certain body weight, at which we
neither gain nor lose weight. The DCML is in the range of
from 1,300 calories (a small, older, inactive person) to 3,000 or
more calories (a large, young, and physically active person).

Since so many factors determine a person's DCML, it therefore is totally incorrect to state (as is often done in diet books)
that a person of a certain age, height, and sex has a daily
caloric requirement of x calories. For example, two women,
Anne and Susan, both 5'4" tall and 24 years old, might find in
some weight-loss charts that their metabolism is 2,300 calories per day. If both women would adjust their food intake to
2,300 calories, Anne would gain weight, but Susan would lose
weight. Why?

Because these numbers are just averages, and they didn't
take into account that Susan is a physically active member of
a neighborhood sports team, whereas Anne has a desk job

with little or no activity at all; Anne prefers reading to exercising and often is the first one to feel cold (an indication of low metabolism, or a below-average number of sodium-potassium pumps in her body.)

It should therefore be quite obvious that weight loss must have a very personalized approach. Learning how to sense what your body needs, or what is bad for it and what to avoid, will help to make this approach a perfect one for you.

1,300 cal/day	*2,200 cal/day*	*3,900 cal/day*
Small person, desk job. No physical-activity program.	Moderately active during day. Minor recreational physical activities.	Heavy laborer. Active member of a neighborhood football team.

No matter what our personal DCML is, about 3,500 calories are equivalent to one pound of extra body weight (fat). The only thing that is different from one person to another is how the weight-loss factors affect the burning of the calories (how your metabolism works). Although one set of weight-loss factors will make it easier for one person to lose weight, a totally different set of factors will do the trick for another person. Doing it wrong can greatly induce premature aging, and doing it right will increase longevity and eliminate many causes of aging.

Make a deal with yourself and set a goal

Your absolute first step in shedding pounds is to set a goal for yourself. But be reasonable! A healthy and lasting weight loss should not exceed three to five pounds per week, depending on body weight and biochemical individuality.

There are fifty ways to leave a lover, and there are at least nine ways to get rid of unwanted pounds. As we discuss the nine weight-loss factors, you will see that most of them can be connected to a certain saving in calories and an equivalent in lost pounds. If you practiced all of them at the same time, you would lose weight far too fast. Once you know which weight-loss factors apply to you, you can choose the ones you like and combine them in a way that fits your life-style and that gives you the desired weight loss.

People often ask us: If I can put on five pounds in three days, why can't I take them off that fast? Compare this to your car: Putting in food is equivalent to filling up the gas tank. You have to drive it quite a distance to burn the fuel. It's the same with your body: You have to move it to burn the calories. Since there is a limit to burning off calories, you must recognize that you have a certain responsibility to your body by not putting in more fuel than you can burn.

After you have determined how many pounds to lose and at what speed you will lose this weight, start thinking about a reward—something you'd really like to have, something you will give yourself when you reach your ideal weight. You don't have to decide right now; we'll tell you more about rewarding yourself with noncaloric items in a later chapter.

You'll also need to make a deal with yourself: Promise yourself that this time you *will* do it, and you *will* go the distance! If it gets a little difficult, we'll find a way to make it easier. Promise yourself at least three weeks on our program. You'll see by then that it really can work.

You'll also learn why two women who are exactly alike in weight, height, and anything you can think of, can be given the same diet to lose weight, and one of them will not shed an ounce. Taking into account the factor that causes this (chapter 9) means accounting for your biochemical individuality.

Does every "overweight" person have to lose weight?

We hear so often that weight loss should be the number one priority for most Americans. Wouldn't *any* weight loss be considered healthy?

Not at all! There are definitely a few people who are probably healthier with a few extra pounds on their bones. And there are those who repeatedly go on some of those ridiculous weight-loss binges and end up putting the weight back on: this extreme does more damage to their bodies than you can imagine. The emphasis should always be on "a permanent and healthy weight loss."

Maybe we should start by defining health. What is health? A dictionary might define it as the "absence of the symptoms of a disease."

This is not entirely true. At first the body gets sick, and then the symptoms appear. Although many diseases have symptoms that show up immediately, there are others that have no symptoms, or the symptoms only show up when the disease is already at a critical stage.

Let me give you an example that is weight related. Thousands of American young men fought in the Korean War. They had passed their physicals and were classified as "healthy." After some of them died in battle, doctors took a look at their arteries and found that many of these young men had atherosclerosis (the narrowing of the arteries that leads to heart attacks). Overweight and lack of exercise are two of the strongest risk factors for atherosclerosis. But these men were not overweight, and they certainly were kept physically active during their military service. Yet, they had this disease even though they were classified as "healthy." It was later found that the wrong overall composition of one's diet and a number of missing vitamins and minerals bring on atherosclerosis. While an inadequate diet brought on the disease in many soldiers, some of them—due to their having the right biochemical makeup—were able to maintain good health.

As you probably know, a higher heart disease risk also means a shorter life span. In separate animal studies, the vitamins and minerals that were lacking in the diet of the soldiers were shown to increase life spans and delay the onset of atherosclerosis.

In holistic and preventive medicine, we define health as "the absence of disease and being able to function at one's optimum possible capacity." According to this definition, being overweight might be classified as a disease because overweight people do not function at optimum capacity, and they often have symptoms indicating a number of other disorders such as depression, high blood pressure, and hypoglycemia.

It's all right to get rid of any extra pounds, but let's do it safely and with common sense. Let's do it with the right nutrition so that we don't age our bodies with unnecessary distress.

Let's do it with the appropriate nutritional supplements to avoid the typical weight-loss, diet-related nutritional deficiencies.

Let's do it with the correct "minimum-effort-for-best-results" physical activities that will help us reduce heart disease risks at the same time.

And let's do it without the ignorance expressed in many diet books:

> "Protein and lots of water"—equals extreme nutritional ignorance.
>
> "Grapefruit only"—staying on this diet for an extended period is just a little bit slower than killing a person with a gun.
>
> "No carbohydrates"—can induce the symptoms of diabetes.
>
> "Low protein"—can induce depression and mental disorders.
>
> "The Cambridge Diet"—can lead to numerous future health risks.

Do you get the picture? Don't cheat your body just to lose a few quick pounds that don't stay off—and that are not worth the health problems they may induce.

Are you willing to work a little bit for a perfect body and excellent health? You must have recognized that our program isn't the Wham-Bang-Five-Pounds-Thank-You-Madam Diet. We make bodies the honest way: You get the body you work for, but it will be a healthy one and it will last.

At this point it is also important to have a talk with your mate or the people you live with. Explain to them that you are going on a weight-loss program and that you'd like their support. This support can come in many forms: by not eating high-calorie foods in front of you; by taking you for a long walk instead of to a bar; or by taking you to dinner at a place where they serve healthy low-calorie foods (see examples in chapter 3, Tables 3.1 and 3.2, and chapter 18) instead of feeding you an all-American monstrous dinner late at night.

Diet pills are a no-no in our approach. They have dangerous side effects that affect your mind and body, and professionals actually feel that they only make a weight problem worse. They might help you a little bit in shedding a few pounds, but as soon as you go back to eating normally, the pounds go on even faster! And if you are not yet convinced, ask your pharmacist for the drug sheets of the two major diet drugs. Read the risks and side effects. I hope it will scare the living h--- out of you.

In holistic and preventive medicine we look at a body and determine what caused it to get sick, and then we make it healthy by giving it what it's missing. By using this line of thinking, can you determine if your weight-problem was brought on by a "diet-pill deficiency"? Naturally not!

Aging isn't just looking older; it can mean getting better

In the popular literature, in movies, and on TV shows, aging is often depicted as one process, and the Frankenstein-type scientist rejuvenates the patients by applying one potion.

The truth can't be further removed from this simple-minded interpretation. There is one thing gerontologists, researchers in the field of aging, agree on: There are at least one hundred more- or less-severe factors that affect the overall speed of the entire aging process. It is the wrong application of most of these factors that usually causes accelerated (or premature) aging; the correct application can delay it.

Many of these factors also contribute to the onset or prevention of specific diseases. An increase in the risk factors for specific diseases also means an increase in the overall rate of aging. We often hear health professionals talk about the "average" human life span. If we could eliminate some of the risk factors for a specific disease, we would definitely increase the average life span of the entire population in a small way, but if we could totally eliminate a disease—for example, cancer—the average life span would greatly increase. As you will see throughout the chapters of this book, even if you have neglected yourself all your life, many of the risk factors can be reversed.

In aging research we talk about the true causes of aging. Many theories on aging have postulated specific causes of aging. Some theories on aging have already died of old age themselves because neither animal experiments nor human studies could confirm the postulated causes; other theories survived and became stronger because interfering with the postulated causes of aging increased the life span of animals and humans.

The disease researchers talk about "disease risks," whereas the gerontologists talk about the "true causes of aging." In many cases we are talking about the same thing. Animal experiments demonstrate that if we apply physical activity the wrong way, it becomes a stress factor causing a shorter life span in the animals. However, if we apply it correctly, a great increase in the average life span will result. It has also been shown that a group of compounds known as *antioxidants* (specific vitamins and minerals) have caused excellent life-span increases in animals. Upon closer examination of the data, we also find that these antioxidants help prevent the onset of diseases such as cancer, heart ailment, and possibly others. Also, remember that being overweight is one of the greatest disease-risk factors that also shortens your life span by nine to fourteen years.

The entire rate of aging is determined by a combination of factors that affect the onset of diseases *and* the true causes of aging. People often feel that the prevention of the so-called "old-age" diseases merely means dragging on for a few more years. They associate being old and living longer with all the negative aspects of old age, such as being incapacitated, looking old, being senile, being impotent, and so forth. They don't understand that practicing the wrong health habits and that ignoring the causes of aging will increase the entire rate of aging and will make them feel and look old at an even earlier stage in life. The gerontologist is well aware of the 40-year-old who has not taken care of his health and who looks 65, and the health-oriented 65-year-old who looks 40.

Aging can be summed up by explaining the longevity studies that were performed in our laboratory. A large number (more than one thousand) Swiss albino mice—prone to cancer just as humans are—were divided into three groups. One group was the "control," and everything these animals received was raised under "standard" conditions. The second group was subjected to all the mistakes people often make: following a diet high in sugar, not exercising, inhaling cigarette smoke, drinking tap water, and not taking vitamin supplements. Group 3 received all of the life-extending factors as suggested by the theories on aging (chapter 16), exercise wheels were installed in their cages, and they were not subjected to negative factors such as a wrong diet or cigarette smoke.

The data showed that the average life span of the animals in group 3 was close to 100 percent longer than in group 2. Animals in group 2 looked older sooner, and their reproductive capacity ceased at a younger age. The life span of group 1 was the midpoint of that for groups 2 and 3.

Therefore, we concluded that aging can be delayed by reaching and maintaining a normal weight and by removing disease risks from your life.

NOW LET'S EVALUATE YOUR METABOLISM

At a party a girl complained to a friend who was gorging herself on a big piece of pizza: "This isn't fair! You can eat anything without gaining weight, and I get fat by merely looking at food."

How often have you heard similar statements? It is quite true that some people burn calories the way race cars burn gasoline, whereas others get fat on a fraction of these calories. We all understand that a number of factors play a role here, but there is one major difference: It is the rate (the speed) of their metabolism.

"I have a slow metabolism," is the usual remark from somebody who just gained some weight. Well, we all need a good excuse for something for which we don't want to take the responsibility, but in this case there is a scientific basis for this phenomenon.

People can have different metabolisms. People with a fast metabolism burn calories easily; they always seem to have some extra energy, and their chances of putting on weight are reduced. People with a slow metabolism often feel cold, and their extra calories are stored as fat rather than burned.

To illustrate this, think of two automobile engines of approximately the same size. One is a high-compression race-car engine, designed to race at top speeds; the other belongs in an economy-car category, designed to go a long distance on a little bit of fuel. Each one has an advantage and disadvantage. When gasoline is cheap, you may want to drive the fast car; but when there is a gasoline crisis, the economy engine is appreciated.

If your metabolism is slow, complaining won't do any good but taking the right action will allow you to take charge of the problem. The trick here is to take charge of the problem the right way, the one that makes it easy for you to shed those pounds. So many people are doing it the wrong way, making weight loss difficult or even impossible. You need to plan for it with your type of metabolism in mind. Therefore, it is important that we take a look at the factors that determine your metabolism.

Sodium-potassium pumps and your metabolism

Mineral and nutrient transport in our body is a very important function. From the digestive tract to the blood, and in the many different types of cells, nutrients and oxidation products are constantly being transported across membranes. This just doesn't happen by itself; it takes energy to do all this. A fireplace in your home can warm the entire room when you burn coal or wood in it; but it also takes some energy to bring the coal and wood into the house and, later, to clean up and remove the ashes.

Very much simplified, this transporting is done in our body by a system consisting of two minerals: sodium and potassium. In our body, most sodium is found outside the cells, and most potassium is found inside the cells. It is believed that nutrients hitch a ride, kind of like a piggyback, on minerals as they pass in and out of the cells.

A number of scientists believe that the system that involves sodium and potassium, called the sodium-potassium pumps, contributes to the determination of a person's metabolism. Some people have fewer than average sodium-potassium pumps, and therefore, they have a lower metabolism. It is also believed that people with fewer sodium-potassium pumps are the ones who often feel cold and are the first ones to put on a sweater if it gets a little cold. Does that description fit you?

Lean muscle mass and your metabolism

The most basic factor that determines how fast or slow your basal metabolism is, is the fat-free body mass or the amount of lean muscle mass on your body. The more muscle mass you have, the higher your basal metabolism. Basal metabolism is defined as the number of calories you burn at rest, without doing anything. For example, Tom, who weighs 180 pounds, was found to have a lower metabolism that Peter, who weighs only 160 pounds. This was explained by a body-composition analysis that showed that Tom had lots of fat on his body, and his total amount of muscle mass was less than Peter's.

At the 1984 meeting of the American College of Sports Medicine, researchers explained their experiments demonstrating the connection between fat-free lean muscle mass and metabolism. They had designed a totally insulated suit— it looked like a space suit—that allowed them to exactly measure the energy expended by a person. Nothing, not body type, not being classified as a "fast" or "slow" oxidizer, nor anything else, affected the rate of their subjects metabolism. What did affect their metabolism was the amount of lean muscle mass they had. The more muscle mass, the higher their metabolism. As a result of these findings, the researchers suggested that only two things determine a person's caloric expenditure: the amount of lean muscle mass and how physically active one is.

When it comes to calories, women have a tougher life than men

When we order a meal in a restaurant, the amount of food served is the same for men and women, even though a man weighs approximately one-third more than a woman. Body composition data also show that healthy women have about 3 percent to 5 percent more body fat than men. If restaurants had "man-sized" and "women-sized" meals, women wouldn't be tempted to overeat. It is quite natural that when you pay lots of money for a good meal, you want to eat everything you are given instead of throwing one-third away.

Because women have more body fat, it is much more important for them to count how many calories there are in each meal. Through this knowledge, they can take the right action. But what is the right action to take? How can they increase their metabolism?

Increasing your metabolism

There is nothing that can be done about the number of sodium-potassium pumps in the body. Increasing or decreasing the sodium or potassium intake will change nothing either. However, there is something you can do about the lean muscle mass on your body. You can make certain, through exercise, that you have a good amount of lean muscle mass. This is especially important for women because that's what gives them an attractive, firm shape. Don't worry, exercise won't make women muscular like men; the difference between male and female hormone levels prevents that. Exercise physiologists now recommend that women use exercise machines to maintain a reasonable amount of lean muscle mass. To become truly muscular, women would have to "pump iron" for several hours every day.

The functioning of the thyroid also affects your metabolism, but the number of people who are affected by a thyroid problem is relatively small. In chapter 3 we'll teach you how to calculate your DCML. If this calculated value, when compared to your actual daily caloric intake, doesn't make sense, you might ask your doctor to check your thyroid. The test to do this is very simple and relatively inexpensive. But before you look for such exotic reasons for having a low metabolism, look at the more commonsense causes such as the wrong body composition, imbalances in macronutrients, lack of certain vitamins or minerals, insufficient physical activity, or other causes.

NOW GO TO FIGURE 10.1 IN CHAPTER 10 AND CHECK ITEM 1

From what you have learned in this chapter, how would you classify your metabolism? The answers to questions such as: Do you often feel cold; are you the first one to put on a sweater? and How much muscle mass do you have on your body? will help you arrive at an answer.

Is a low metabolism indicated? If yes, check item 1a— "Activate lean muscle mass with exercise" in Figure 10.1.

As we said before, it is possible that you have a low thyroid function, but before you run to your doctor, make sure that you are doing everything right as discussed in the first nine chapters. At least, wait until you have read chapter 3.

2

FACTOR #2
YOUR BODY MEASUREMENTS: Needed to demonstrate your body-shaping weight-loss success.

> About the only time overweight will make a
> man feel better is when he sees it on a girl he
> nearly married.
>
> A. O. Battista

CHECK YOURSELF

To pinpoint the best possible approach for a safe and lasting body-shaping weight loss, we have to keep track of weight, body measurements, and possibly even body fat. Seeing these variables change while on your weight-loss program is a revelation to many people; it is the best encouragement to stick to this program.

1. Do you know what your ideal
   weight should be according to
   height and frame-size charts?   YES   NO

2. Can you name the three most
   important measuring sites on your

33

body that will clearly indicate a
weight change.   YES   NO

3. Did you recently have your body
   fat measured, or has any professional examined you and determined that the fat on your body is
   truly in excess of what it should
   be?   YES   NO

If you answered "YES" to all three questions, you can skip
this chapter and check "Already doing" for item 2 in Figure
10.1.

TO SHED OR NOT TO SHED THOSE POUNDS

How much weight would you like to lose? What are your
criteria for determining the optimum weight loss? Do you
want to lose the weight because:

• You would like to fit into a smaller dress size?

• You want to reduce the size of certain body parts, such as
thighs, buttocks, and/or upper arms?

• Your doctor told you to?

• Your lover would like you to be skinny, and you figured
that this specific weight loss would do it?

All of the above reasons can be wrong. During a medical
meeting, a weight-loss professional gave three examples of
why the above reasons may not be right for you:

1. Two women, 5 feet 6 inches tall, weighed the same: 139
pounds. After an examination, one woman was told to lose
about 15 pounds, while the other was told she should definitely not lose any weight but could even gain some weight.

Explanation: The first woman had a small frame size and
the other one had a large frame size. Using weight and frame
tables, as we will explain shortly, is a safe starting point for
determining a safe weight loss.

2. Again, two women, both weighing 139 pounds, and both

5 feet 6 inches tall, were evaluated regarding the need for weight loss. Both were found to have a medium frame size, and their actual weight was within desired ranges for their body frames. After measuring their body fat, one was advised to lose about six pounds, whereas the other was advised to maintain her weight.

Explanation: Even though both women were within desired weight ranges, according to weight and frame charts, their body fat was quite different. One had an excess of body fat, the other had better muscle tone, due to lots of physical activity, and was on the low side of body-fat ranges.

3. Another set of two women with the same weight and height (139 pounds, 5 feet 6 inches tall) were found to fit normal ranges of weight and frame-size charts, and their body fat was also acceptable. Yet, they were unhappy with their individual weight. One was allowed to shed just a few (up to four) pounds, and she was advised to do leg exercises and some serious jogging. The other woman was told to maintain her weight and to do, in addition to her daily jogging, a number of chest and arm exercises.

Explanation: Their body types were different. Minor differences in body structure, which can easily be corrected with specific exercises, can give the impression that body weight is not normal. For the first woman, a slight weight loss and leg exercises reduced the size of her buttocks and thighs. Leg and buttocks measurements were fine for the other woman, but her chest and bust line were small. The arm and chest exercises increased her upper body measurements, and her overall body appearance was improved. This type of body shaping usually uses specific exercises, but in some cases, surgical techniques may be used (see chapter 7).

What is your body type? What is your frame size, and what is the percentage of fat on your body? Determine your frame and weight range by checking Table 2.1. For the best health, stay on the low end of your weight range or slightly below it.

Now, decide: How much weight should you lose?

Table 2.1
1983 METROPOLITAN HEIGHT AND WEIGHT TABLES

Men

Feet	Inches	Small frame	Medium frame	Large frame
5	3	130-136	133-143	140-153
5	4	132-138	135-145	142-156
5	5	134-140	137-148	144-160
5	6	136-142	139-151	146-164
5	7	138-145	142-154	149-168
5	8	140-148	145-157	152-172
5	9	142-151	148-160	155-176
5	10	144-154	151-163	158-180
5	11	146-157	154-166	161-184
6	0	149-160	157-170	164-188
6	1	152-164	160-174	168-192
6	2	155-168	164-178	172-197
6	3	158-172	167-182	176-202

Women

Feet	Inches	Small frame	Medium frame	Large frame
4	11	103-113	111-123	120-134
5	0	104-115	113-126	122-137
5	1	106-118	115-129	125-140
5	2	108-121	118-132	128-143
5	3	111-124	121-135	131-147
5	4	114-127	124-138	134-151
5	5	117-130	127-141	137-155
5	6	120-133	130-144	140-159
5	7	123-136	133-147	143-163
5	8	126-139	136-150	146-167
5	9	129-142	139-153	149-170
5	10	132-145	142-156	152-173
5	11	135-148	145-159	155-176

Courtesy of the Metropolitan Life Insurance Company.

Note: From the *Metropolitan Life Insurance Company,* the above data is based on a new study of the effects of weight on longevity. People at these weights lived longer than people who weighed more. This newly revised table recommends slightly higher weight levels than earlier tables. Nevertheless, recent studies suggest that staying at the *low end* of the recommended levels is still the healthiest choice. A number of gerontologists and health professionals believe that the ideal weight is 10 percent below these ranges.

WEIGHING YOURSELF

"Don't ask me to get on a scale. I could never face those numbers," is a statement we hear from many people.

But by buying this book you have already taken the first step toward losing those extra pounds. It is only by weighing yourself that you will be able to appreciate your weight-loss success. Getting on a scale every day and seeing your weight drop will encourage you to stick to this program. And of course, you must weigh yourself in order to find out how much to lose to see how fast you are shedding the pounds and, also, to make sure you are not losing weight too fast.

Always weigh yourself in the morning, right after you get up. Don't be afraid of the bathroom scale. After a short time on this program, it will only give you good news in the morning, and you will also learn to recognize when you have made mistakes. Variations in your weight during the day (due to activities, food and fluid intake, and bowel movements) can be as much as several pounds, which is the reason for weighing yourself in the morning.

Every second day, record your weight on the chart (Fig. 2.1) provided. If you don't want anybody to see it just copy the chart (squared graph paper makes it easier to record) and place it in a safe and convenient place.

The vertical subdivisions represent one pound each. Record your present weight on the highest mark. Each subdivision on the horizontal line represents one day. Mark the date when you start your program. Then, as you weigh yourself, make a

Figure 2.1. Your Personal Weight-Loss Chart. Charting your weight is not a requirement for our program, but it will certainly help.

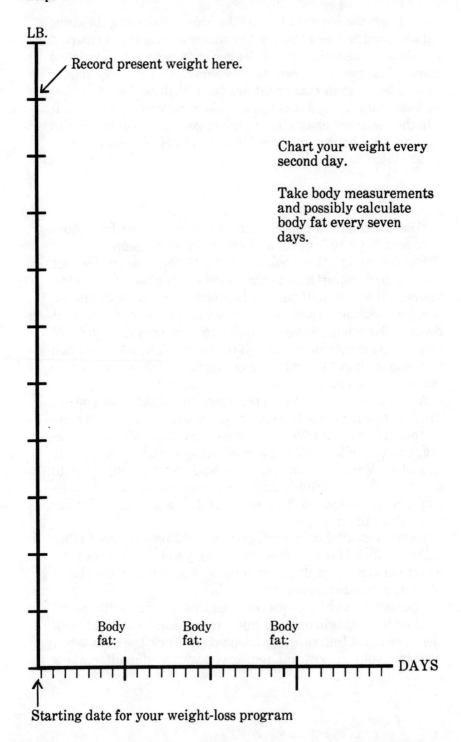

check mark above the date that corresponds to your weight. This chart is important. If you do things right, it will result in a downward curve. If you can lose five pounds in two weeks, you will lose ten pounds in one month, and so on.

This chart will also take the mystery out of your weight loss. By keeping track of what you are doing, you will see which weight-loss factors are truly effective for you, and you will also recognize your mistakes.

OTHER WEIGHT-RELATED BODY MEASUREMENTS

How often have you heard someone say, "Not only did I lose weight, but more important, I lost inches and got into shape!" Well, that's what this program is all about.

Depending on what kind of physical condition you are in, there might be a short time when your weight loss comes to a halt. This could be because you are losing fat but you are also building important lean muscle tissue. When people watch only their weight, they might be discouraged at this point. However, if they can see how their measurements are improving, they won't give up.

Figure 2.2 shows how to measure your body—take your measurements, record them at the bottom of the page, remeasure every seven days. These same measurements can also be used to calculate your body fat. Body fat is a good indicator of how much weight to lose.

There are also a number of people who just feel fat because of an uneven distribution of fat on their body; for them, body shaping together with weight loss would give the best possible results. And then, there are people who are so obsessed with losing weight that they go to extremes and become anorexic. Measuring body fat could prevent these people from making serious mistakes.

Accepted ranges of body fat are from 13 percent to 18· percent for men and from 16 percent to 23 percent for women. Athletes are, on an average, 2 percent below these limits.

Figure 2.2. How to Measure Your Body. The sites shown are good indicators for weight loss or weight gain.

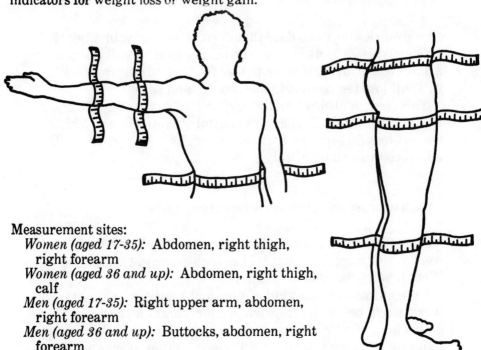

Measurement sites:
Women (aged 17-35): Abdomen, right thigh, right forearm
Women (aged 36 and up): Abdomen, right thigh, calf
Men (aged 17-35): Right upper arm, abdomen, right forearm
Men (aged 36 and up): Buttocks, abdomen, right forearm

In measuring, follow these guidelines:
Abdomen: ½ inch above the navel
Buttocks: maximum protrusion with heels together
Right thigh: upper thigh just below the buttocks
Right upper arm: arm straight, palm out and extended in front of the body (measure midway between the shoulder and the elbow)
Right forearm: widest circumference, between the elbow and the wrist
Right calf: widest circumference midway between the ankle and the knee

Your measurements (three sites, taken every seven days):

Date:	Date:	Date:
1)	1)	1)
2)	2)	2)
3)	3)	3)

Body fat can be measured

Underwater weighing compares your actual weight to your weight when immersed in water. This is a very good method for measuring body fat, but it must be done by an expert; also, it is not available everywhere.

Skin-fold measurements can be made with a number of devices. Using skin-fold calipers, a number of different skin-fold thicknesses can be determined. When the data are plugged into a formula and a few simple calculations are made, you have your body-fat percentage.

Another easy method to check your body fat was developed by Drs. Frank Katch and William McArdle; it uses the same three body measurements as in Figure 2.2. Again, plugging the numbers into a simple formula allows you to calculate your body-fat percentage. If you want to calculate your body fat yourself, go to the library and check out *Getting In Shape* by Drs. Katch and McArdle. The procedure is easy to follow, and since you already have your measurements, it will take only a few minutes to arrive at an answer.

Your body composition can be measured by electrical impedance. A device developed by RJL Systems of Detroit measures electrical impedance by placing two electrodes on different parts of your body. The entire procedure takes only about five minutes and the computer readout gives you the percentage of body fat, total amount of fat in pounds, total lean body weight, and much more. (You'll find the address of RJL Systems in the References.)

You can get your body fat measured without charge. A number of health clubs use this method. We've made an agreement with the health clubs listed in Appendix B at the back of this book. They will measure your body fat for free when you come in for a first (also free) visit. Just bring this book along and show it to them but call ahead of time for an appointment.

When measuring your body, fat becomes very important. When you get close to your ideal weight, when you are not sure if you should lose a few more pounds, when you work hard on losing pounds and are not successful, then measuring the percentage of fat on your body becomes important. If you are already in the desired range, don't push it too far; going to extremes can be very harmful to your health.

Not very long ago, when I was involved in a strong interval training program, my body fat was measured at 13.8 percent. I was going very strong and wondered if reducing my body fat to 9 percent would make me feel even better. After I did so, I realized something was wrong. I couldn't pinpoint the trouble, but I surely wasn't feeling so great. So, with the help of a friend of mine, a doctor who specialized in preventive medicine, we determined a number of tests, including blood and urine analysis, and found that several health factors were outside the accepted ranges. Everything returned to normal when I allowed my body fat to return to my original range of from 13 percent to 14 percent.

It is also possible for a person of "normal" weight (according to the weight tables), or for someone who looks skinny, to have a very high percentage of body fat. This is the case with people who have very little muscle mass; their body tissues feel soft and spongy. For these people to get an *exact* measure of body fat, one has to use the underwater-weighing technique or the RJL method.

Measuring your body fat is not an absolute requirement for our weight-loss program, but we recommend it since you will have a much better idea about where you stand, what has to be done, and how far you have to go.

NOW GO TO FIGURE 10.1 AND CHECK ITEM 2

1. Be sure to weigh yourself every morning, right after you get up, and record your weight every second day in your weight-loss chart.

2. Take the three body measurements, as shown in Figure 2.2 every seven days.

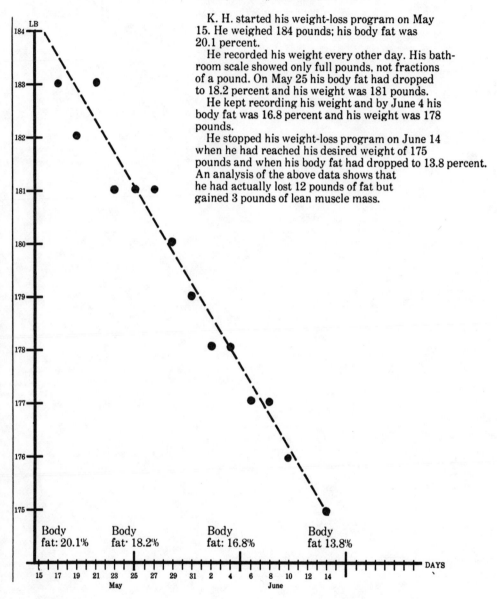

Example. Weight-Loss Chart

K. H. started his weight-loss program on May 15. He weighed 184 pounds; his body fat was 20.1 percent.

He recorded his weight every other day. His bathroom scale showed only full pounds, not fractions of a pound. On May 25 his body fat had dropped to 18.2 percent and his weight was 181 pounds.

He kept recording his weight and by June 4 his body fat was 16.8 percent and his weight was 178 pounds.

He stopped his weight-loss program on June 14 when he had reached his desired weight of 175 pounds and when his body fat had dropped to 13.8 percent. An analysis of the above data shows that he had actually lost 12 pounds of fat but gained 3 pounds of lean muscle mass.

Figure 2.3

3

FACTOR #3

SUPERNUTRITION—A Two-Part Event: The result of caloric content and the quality of your food.

> WEIGHT LOSS WOULD BE EASY IF SPARE PARTS WEREN'T AVAIL-ABLE IN THE REFRIGERATOR.
> Caption from poster by the
> Spenco Medical Corporation

CHECK YOURSELF

An introduction to applied supernutrition covers two areas. First, we determine how many calories you can consume per day without gaining weight and adjust this DCML downward to guarantee a weight loss. Second, we teach you a little bit of nutrition and make sure that the calories are consumed in terms of quality foods and in the right proportion. Faulty nutrition is a major factor in heart disease, diabetes, and cancer.

1. Do you know how many calories you would have to consume per day in order to maintain your ideal body weight?   YES   NO

2. Do you know what your actual
   average daily caloric intake is?   YES   NO

3. Do you know how many calories
   are equivalent to one pound of fat?   YES   NO

4. Quickly go to Tables 3.1–3.3 in this
   chapter. Is your daily food intake
   reasonably close to what we
   recommend?   YES   NO

If you answered "YES" to all four questions, you can skip
this chapter and check "Already doing" for item 3 in Figure
10.1. But before you move on to the next chapter, check your
answers to item 1 and 4 to make sure that they are correct.

CALORIES AND WEIGHT LOSS

Before we start our discussion of supernutrition, let's just
make sure that you understand the connection between calories and weight loss or weight gain, as demonstrated in Figure 3.1.

The DCML is the daily caloric intake level at which you
neither gain nor lose weight. If you consume more calories
than the DCML, you gain weight; if you consume less, you lose
weight.

Approximately 3,500 calories are equivalent to one pound
of extra body weight (fat). If a person consumes 500 calories
more every day than one's DCML, this amounts to a weight
gain of one pound per week (500 times 7, divided by 3,500).
Consuming 500 calories less than the DCML gives a weight
loss of one pound per week, or four pounds per month. Twice
this caloric reduction leads to a loss of two pounds per week, or
eight pounds per month.

In general:

$$\begin{array}{l} \text{daily caloric} \\ \text{reduction below} \\ \text{the DCML} \end{array} \times 7 \div 3{,}500 = \begin{array}{l} \text{weight loss} \\ \text{in pounds} \\ \text{per week} \end{array}$$

Figure 3.1. The Connection Between Weight and Food Intake.
Effect of calories consumed:
1. If you consume fewer calories than
   the DCML, a weight loss should (and
   often will) result.
2. If you consume more calories than
   the Daily Caloric Maintenance Level
   (DCML), a weight gain will result.

CALORIC INTAKE
(with everything else
remaining the
same):

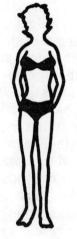

If caloric
intake is
decreased

DCML

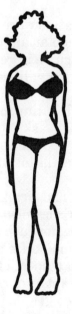

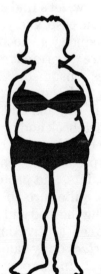

If caloric
intake is
increased

THERE IS A LIMIT TO CALORIC REDUCTIONS

Since we must maintain a minimum caloric intake to assure good health, and since caloric reductions make you hungry all the time, there is a definite limit to weight loss through caloric reductions.

Doesn't everybody who wants to lose weight have to eat less? Not at all! That idea is a typical diet-book concept. There are many overweight people who exist on a minimum-calorie diet and telling them to eat even less would be highly irresponsible. Their weight problems can be solved by other measures.

For other people it might be sufficient to switch to different types of foods that will increase the volume of foods consumed but not the total caloric content. And, believe it or not, there are even a number of people for whom we will advise an increase in food intake in combination with a change to different food groups.

All this depends very much on what you are presently eating. Are you a junk-food junky? A vegetarian? On a high- or low-protein diet? We will discuss nutrition in general and, by comparing it to your present diet, you will learn which changes are right for you.

For now, let's find out if you are simply eating too much. If this is the case, and you worry that I might ask you to drastically reduce your food intake, relax! As I pointed out earlier, there are ways to eat more while reducing the total number of calories consumed.

Step 1: Keep track of what you eat and drink during a "typical" day and add up all the calories consumed. Get yourself a notebook and keep a nutritional log; for each day, count all the calories and the grams of protein and fat consumed. The types of foods and their content in respect of carbohydrates, fats, and proteins are unimportant as of now. If you are not quite sure about the numbers you get, do it again by recalling the food and drinks you consumed yesterday, or do it for two consecutive days and average out the numbers. This is your *actual* daily caloric intake.

Step 2: In chapter 2, you determined, from the weight-height tables, your ideal weight in pounds. If you are 34 or younger, multiply your ideal weight by 15. If you are 35 or older, multiply your ideal weight by 13. This gives you your daily caloric maintenance level, the number of calories required per day to maintain this body weight. This number includes a reasonable amount of physical activity.

$$\underline{\hspace{3cm}} \times \underline{\hspace{5cm}} = \underline{\hspace{2cm}}$$

Ideal weight   15 (if 34 yrs. or younger)   DCML
13 (if 35 yrs. or older)

If you determined earlier (in chapter 1) that you had a slow metabolism, subtract approximately 150 calories from this calculated DCML. This will mostly be for people who have a high amount of body fat or very little lean muscle mass. *On this new, adjusted DCML you will definitely not gain any weight. You might even lose some weight.*

Step 3: Compare your actual daily caloric intake (step 1) to your calculated DCML. If the number is higher than the calculated value, then it is obvious that you eat too much (in terms of calories). Don't worry if caloric reductions are difficult for you; later, we will show you how to deal with this problem. If your actual daily caloric intake is about the same as the calculated DCML, or even lower, be careful not to make extreme caloric reductions; as you will see in later chapters, your weight problem might be caused by other factors such as the sugar in your diet, insufficient physical activity, or a number of other factors.

How much could you, should you, reduce calories?

Health experts agree that we should never dip below 800 calories per day for a small and inactive person; 900 calories for a medium-weight and fairly active person; and 1,000 calories for a larger or more active person.

In order to achieve a maximum weight loss, one could lower the caloric intake down to the minimum level. Many diet books make this recommendation—and fail. Why? Because such extreme caloric restrictions are easier to recommend than to follow. People start with good intentions, but when they find themselves under stress because the diet is difficult to maintain, they soon give up.

DETERMINING YOUR DESIRED (FEASIBLE) DAILY CALORIC INTAKE

In order to make a weight-loss program work, we must arrive at a daily caloric intake that you can live with and that will also give you the desired weight loss. We therefore let you determine your daily caloric intake. It must, however, be somewhere between your absolute minimum level and calculated DCML. We suggest that you start with a daily caloric intake that is halfway between these two values. If you find this easy to do, you can always lower your caloric intake a little bit more later on.

Example: A 26-year-old woman determines from the weight-height tables that her ideal weight should be 105 pounds. Her calculated DCML therefore is 105 times 15, which is 1,575 calories. Since she is a small and relatively inactive person, her minimum daily caloric intake must be at least 800 calories. A good starting point for her would be around 1,200 calories per day, which is halfway between 800 calories and 1,575 calories.

Record your calculated DCML and your desired daily caloric intake in your weight-loss chart in chapter 2 and, also, in your food log.

At this point you know approximately how many calories you can have in your daily diet. Our next step is to teach you about nutrition so that the calories you ingest are derived from quality foods and so that the amounts of nutrients such as carbohydrates, fats, and proteins are in the right range.

LEARNING MORE ABOUT NUTRITION

Don't worry! I'm not going to try to make a health-food nut out of you.

This chapter on supernutrition is designed to give you a

basic understanding of how carbohydrates, fats, proteins, vitamins, and minerals interact in your body to make up the most perfect nutrition for you. Knowing what certain food groups do for your body will also give you an idea of what can go wrong in your body if you omit certain foods from your diet, or how weight is put on if the ratio of foods is not correct, or if you just eat too much of one specific food.

For a better understanding of nutrition, take a quick look at the foods in Tables 3.1–3.2, so that you know which foods are "desirable" and which ones are "undesirable." You could photocopy these tables and carry them with you when you grocery shop or eat out. By following the amounts of foods recommended in Tables 3.1 and 3.2 you will have an 800-calories- to 900-calories-per-day intake. Add more foods to bring *your* intake to the desired calorie level.

SUPERNUTRITION FOR SUPERBODIES

For the following discussion of the nutrients in our foods, and what happens to them in our body, use Figure 3.2 to get a good overview of the pathways they take in a body that functions normally. The wrong food supply and faulty health practices can greatly alter the entire picture, and it will become clear to you why you should follow our nutritional advice.

In Praise of Protein
Protein is broken down (digested) by the body into amino acids, the basic building-block units. As far as weight control is concerned, the most important function of amino acids is to build muscle mass. Other functions are to form enzymes, repair body tissues (such as skin, hair, and nails), and keep the nervous system sparking normally. A body lacking just a small amount of protein can affect any one of these functions. Since the body has almost no storage capacity for amino acids, except in a process known to the biochemist as *compartmentation*, we want to eat a slight excess of protein at regular intervals. Any excess of amino acids is burned to give energy.

Table 3.1
Complex Carbohydrates

Vegetables and Grains

Include two to three portions of these foods and spices per day. You can eat these foods in very liberal amounts (except if noted as occasional). The caloric content will range from 20 to 50 calories per cup.

Liberal		*Occasional*
Alfalfa sprouts	Gelatin (unsweetened)	Artichokes
Beans, green	Kale	Barley
Beet greens	Kohlrabi	Brown rice
Beets, red	Lemons	Bulgur
Broccoli	Lettuce	Corn
Brussels sprouts	Limes	Millet
Cabbage	Mung bean sprouts	Peas
Capers	Mushrooms	Potatoes
Carrots	Okra	Sweet potatoes
Cauliflower	Onions	
Celery	Parsley	
Chard	Pepper, black	
Chicory greens	Pepper, green or red	
Chili peppers	Pickles (unsweetened)	
Chinese cabbage	Pimientos	
Chives	Radishes	
Clam juice	Rhubarb (unsweetened)	
Collard greens	Romaine	
Cranberries	Sauerkraut	
(unsweetened)	Scallions	
Cucumbers	Snap beans	
Curry powder	Soybean sprouts	
Dandelion greens	Spices	
Dill	Spinach	
Dill pickles (unsweetened)	Summer squash	
Duruka (Fiji asparagus)	Taro leaves	

Egg plant
Endive
Escarole
Fennel

Tomatoes
Truffles
Turnip greens
Watercress

Fruits

Include two servings of any unsweetened fruit per day (except if noted as occasional). The caloric content is from 60 to 100 calories per serving.

Two servings	*Occasional* *(½ or small portion)*
Apples	Avocado
Apricots	Banana
Berries (all, ½ C)	Cherries
Cantaloupe	Figs
Grapefruit	Grapes
Oranges	Honeydew
Papaya (small)	Kumquats
Peaches	Mango
Plums	Pear
Tangerines	Pineapple
Watermelon (sm. pcs.)	Pomegranate
	Prunes

Breads and Cereals

With every meal, include one portion of the following bread or cereal foods. Butter may be used very sparingly. Read the label of your bread products to make sure that no sugar has been added.

1 slice of any high-quality bread—whole-grain, nine-grain, protein, or high-fiber bread (40–60 cal, fiber).

1 bran muffin; homemade or bought at health store. Read the label for sugar; honey is preferred (80 cal, fiber).

½ English muffin—whole wheat (60 cal, fiber).

½ cup of cold cereal; no sugar added—corn flakes, wheat flakes, puffed rice, puffed wheat, puffed millet (110 cal, not including milk; fiber).

1/3 cup of hot cereal; no sugar added—cream of wheat, oat bran, oatmeal, corn meal (110 cal, fiber).

½ bagel—whole wheat (60 cal, some fiber).

Table 3.2
Protein Foods

Make sure that each meal includes one portion of any one of the foods listed below (three portions per day). If you are very active and if your ideal weight is over 120 pounds, you can have up to four portions per day.

Non fat milk, 1 cup (90 cal, 9 g protein)
Low-fat milk, 1 cup (130 cal, 9 g protein)
Veal, 3 oz (185 cal, 23 g protein)
Egg, one (80 cal, 6 g protein)
Nuts or seeds, 1 oz, unsalted, raw or dry roasted (180 cal, 6 g
  protein)
Chicken, 3 oz, well done, no fat added, skin removed (115 cal,
  20 g protein)
Nonfat cottage cheese, 3 oz (75 cal, 15 g protein)
Low-fat cheese, 3 oz (100 cal, 9 g protein)
Swiss or cheddar cheese, 1 oz (110 cal, 6 g protein)
Fish, 3 oz broiled or baked (100 cal, 16 g protein)
Lima, kidney, and white beans, 3 oz (110 cal, 12 g protein)
Tofu, 3.5 oz (72 cal, 8 g protein)

Protein insurance: Your daily protein intake should be at least 60 to 100 grams per day, depending on your ideal weight and physical activity. You can assume that you get about 10 grams from the foods in Table 3.1. If you are not eating the protein foods mentioned above on a regular basis (three times per day), then you should have some protein insurance. Get yourself a good protein powder—Octa-protein (available in health-food stores) is an excellent product because it contains octacosanol, an endurance factor. Mix this protein powder with nonfat milk, kefir, or yogurt. You can add a few pieces of fruit for flavoring. Half a glass of this mixture gives you good protein insurance.

Table 3.3
The No-No Foods

Until you have reached your weight goal, avoid the foods listed below. If you find it difficult to eliminate these foods, experiment by eating only half the amount you usually eat and continue decreasing these foods that can interfere with weight loss until you no longer desire them. As you make progress with each chapter, you will find these foods no longer appeal to you.

Sugary Foods	*High-Calorie Foods*
Biscuits	Alcoholic beverages
Brownies	*Avocado
Cake	*Bacon
Candy	*Beans and pork
Cereal, presweetened	Beer
Chewing gum	*Butter
(unless calorie-free)	*Canned meats
Chocolate	*Chili con carne
Cinnamon sugar	*Corned beef
Cookies	*Corn chips
Corn syrup	*Cream
Danish pastry	*Cream cheese
Doughnuts	Cream powder (nondairy creamer)
Fruit canned in syrup	*Cream sauce
Fruit juice, sweetened	*Custard
Honey	*French fries
Ice cream	*Fried chicken
Ice cream soda	*Fried foods, of any sort
Jam	*Hollandaise sauce
Jelly	*Hot dog
Muffins	*Ketchup
Pancakes	*Mayonnaise
Puddings	*Olives

Soft drinks
 (unless calorie-free
Sugar
Syrup, any kind
Waffles

*Olive oil
*Pastrami
*Popcorn, buttered
*Potato chips
 Potato salad
 Pretzels
*Processed meats
*Salad dressings, bottled
*Salami
*Salted nuts
*Sausage
*Steak, marbled
*Tartar sauce
*Whipped cream
*White sauce
*Whole milk

*Contains mostly fats

Proteins should make up from 15 percent to 20 percent of our daily caloric intake. Professor Nevin Scrimshaw, at MIT, demonstrated that as we get older, protein absorption decreases quite a bit, which is why, after the age of 30, we should consume somewhat more protein.

There are about twenty different amino acids, and ten of them are classified as "essential" because the body can't do without them. In general, consuming a cross section of different proteins will supply all the needed amino acids. True vegetarians must supply their bodies with larger amounts of proteins because vegetable proteins are difficult for the body to utilize and they don't supply all the essential amino acids. That's one of the reasons why in nutrition books animal proteins are often referred to as "complete" and individual vegetable proteins as "incomplete."

For people whose blood-sugar level is low, amino acids can be converted into glucose and, thus, help maintain the blood-sugar homeostasis (keeping the blood-sugar level within the right range).

Quality proteins are obtained from lean meats, eggs, low-fat dairy products, fish, fowl, vegetables, nuts, and seeds.

Many weight-loss programs make one major mistake regarding protein intake; they cut down evenly on all calories, including protein, and they increase people's caloric expenditure through exercise—and then they wonder why it is impossible for people in their programs to rebuild lean muscle mass. Because protein needs are directly proportional to the caloric expenditure, protein intake must be slightly increased instead of decreased.

Carbohydrates—good guys and bad guys

Carbohydrates are the main sources of fuel for the body and, when digested, mainly provide us with glucose. An adequate intake of carbohydrates assists in maintaining tissue protein. Also, carbohydrates are needed to more effectively burn off fat. Our central nervous system operates almost exclusively on glucose, and an inadequate amount of carbohydrates severely limits endurance exercise and the functioning of the nervous system.

Sixty percent or more of our daily caloric intake should come from carbohydrates (ideally the unrefined kind). Nutritionists often subdivide carbohydrates into two groups: Natural or "complex" carbohydrates (the good guys), and processed or "refined" carbohydrates (the bad guys). The complex carbohydrates—foods grown and unprocessed—consist of fruits, vegetables, and whole grain products; they are more desirable because they are converted into blood sugar slowly, and they supply us with vitamins, minerals, and roughage.

The refined carbohydrates are essentially high in calories, but low in nutritional value. They include sugar, sweets, soft drinks, white bread, sugary cereals, white flour, and so forth. These empty calories are rapidly converted into glucose, causing blood-sugar imbalances. An excessive consumption of refined carbohydrates has been associated with many medical disorders ranging from tooth decay to diabetes and heart disease.

For weight control, the most important function of carbohydrates is to supply the body with glucose. Glucose is either

Figure 3.2. Normal Pathways of Foods in Your Body.

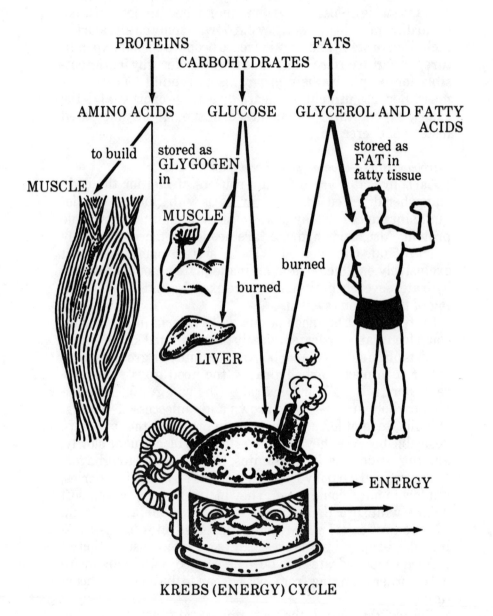

FOOD INTAKE

PROTEINS   FATS

CARBOHYDRATES

AMINO ACIDS   GLUCOSE   GLYCEROL AND FATTY ACIDS

to build   stored as GLYGOGEN in   stored as FAT in fatty tissue

MUSCLE

MUSCLE

burned

LIVER   burned

ENERGY

KREBS (ENERGY) CYCLE

stored in the liver and lean muscle mass as glycogen, or it is burned in the body's furnace (the Krebs Cycle) to give energy. Excess glucose is converted into fat (Fig. 3.2).

Fats—Most people consume far too much
The basic functions of fat are to:
1. provide energy for prolonged physical activities,
2. serve as a cushion for the protection of vital organs,
3. provide insulation from cold, and
4. act as carriers of vitamins A, D, E, and K.

The average American diet gets about 42 percent of its total calories from fat. Experts in the field of heart disease recommend ranges of 10 percent (Pritikin) to 34 percent (Fred Stare, Harvard). However, since Dr. McGee (American Heart Association meeting, 1983) reported that people with a fat intake of less than 25 percent had a higher heart disease and cancer risk, we suggest maintaining the average fat intake at around 25 percent. People who are on a weight-loss program, where some of the fat that is being burned comes from deposited body-fat, can go as low as 20 percent.

It is not good to replace all your fats with polyunsaturates, because increased aging due to free radical formation and a higher cancer risk is definitely associated with a high polyunsaturated diet.

Unsaturated oils from plant sources, such as safflower or corn oil, supply us with "essential" fatty acids and are important for normal hormonal control of the body and for good immune functions. According to Dr. D. Horrobin, approximately 3 to 5 percent of total calories should come from polyunsaturates. Since some very important essential fatty acids are found in Oil of Evening Primrose, which also helps in reducing premenstrual syndrome (PMS), many experts are recommending the use of this oil. A good booklet on this and other important oils by Dr. Jeffrey Bland can be found in health food stores.

There is also a fat-forming enzyme in our bodies that can make you hungry for foods rich in fats. Research data reported during a weight-loss session of the American College of Sports Medicine (San Diego, 1984) showed that the activity of this enzyme is increased by high-fat and extremely low-fat diets, and that it is decreased by a moderate low-fat diet and/or by exercise. Our moderate low-fat approach is therefore supported again.

As for weight control, the two most important reactions in the body are the storage of fat in the adipose tissue and the burning of fat in the incinerator, the Krebs cycle, to give energy. To effectively burn fat, it must be burned together with carbohydrates. If there are no available carbohydrates,. the fat is burned inefficiently, the Krebs cycle doesn't work, and *ketosis* is the end result. Ketosis puts stress on the body; it changes the pH factor and causes excessive urination, which causes minerals to be washed out of the body. Because ketosis is an unhealthy way to lose weight, we want to try hard to prevent it from happening.

Therefore, to effectively control weight we want to supply the body with proteins and complex carbohydrates so that the fat required to make the Krebs cycle (the incinerator) run efficiently is now taken from the stored body fat.

FLUID INTAKE

Depending on weight and physical activity, you should drink from six to eight glasses of water every day. Much of this water can be contained in drinks such as coffee, tea, herbal tea, vegetable or meat broth (homemade or from a health-food store), mineral water, spring water, and fruit juices (unsweetened and or diluted with mineral water).

When we mention coffee as a drink, this doesn't mean that we want you to drink coffee. Coffee, taken black, is just one of those calorie-free fluids. However, we all know about the risks associated with an excessive caffeine intake; so be reasonable in your consumption or drink decaffeinated coffee.

The same reasoning goes for diet drinks. Saccharin is still a cancer risk factor even though a small one. It would be better to try some other calorie-free drinks, such as herbal tea, to keep the overall intake of sweeteners down. If you don't, at least dilute the diet drinks with a good mineral water.

A number of healthy non-caloric fizzes, sweetened with NutraSweet are also available in stores. Some of them, like Vita-Fizz from Nutrition Science Laboratories, are fruit-flavored and contain some vitamins. Just pop one of those tablets into a glass of ice water and you have a delicious drink that is non-caloric, tasty, healthy, and inexpensive.

Tap water, from which most water-based drinks are made, has recently been shown to contain many cancer-causing substances. So-called "health experts" might tell you that "such small quantities are no risk to your health." However, prevention-oriented doctors will disagree with them. The toxic chemicals in the tap water can be removed by attaching a carbon-based filter to your water faucet. These filters are available in every department store, or you can use bottled spring water that has been carbon filtered.

Would you like to know how bad the situation really is? Check the appendix to find out how you can get a free toxic-chemicals report.

All of the chemical reactions in your body, from digesting foods to burning them to making new body tissues, are controlled by enzymes. And that's where vitamins and minerals come in. A complete enzyme is usually made up of a protein that is synthesized by the body and a vitamin or mineral. Naturally vitamins and minerals have many other functions in the body, but in relation to general nutrition, the formation of enzymes is the most important one. We'll learn more about the other functions of vitamins and minerals in chapter 6.

NOW GO TO FIGURE 10.1 AND CHECK ITEM 3

1. Are you already maintaining caloric balance; is your daily caloric intake in the correct range to guarantee weight loss? Do you know your actual daily caloric intake?

2. How good is your nutrition relative to what it should be (Tables 3.1–3.3)? Compare your actual nutrition to our standards and record what, if any, adjustments should be made. No need to be perfect. Make adjustments so that you get a little bit closer to good nutrition.

4

THE SIZE OF YOUR STOMACH—How to prevent hunger with fewer calories

Q.: How long do you eat?
A.: Until I am full.

CHECK YOURSELF

The nutrition guidelines presented in chapter 3 were designed to improve your overall nutrition; they included lowering the amount of fats and increasing the fiber in your diet to bring these two variables within reasonable ranges. For some people, reducing fats and increasing fiber even further, can only have beneficial effects. Large amounts of fiber in the diet help to lower heart disease risk factors such as blood cholesterol and also can eliminate cancer of the colon by up to 95 percent. Excess fat in the diet is also a general cancer risk factor. In addition, lowering the amount of fats and increasing the fiber in your diet helps to fill the stomach and reduce hunger.

1. In comparison to other people, do
   you rate the capacity of your stomach as large (meaning that you
   always have room for more food?   YES   NO
2. Even after following our nutrition
   guidelines in chapter 3, do you still
   feel hungry when you reduce your
   food intake?   YES   NO

If you answered "NO" to both questions, you can check
"Doesn't apply" for item 4 in Figure 10.1 and move on to the
next chapter.

HOW LONG DO YOU EAT?

When you sit down for a meal, when do you quit eating?
When you've had enough? And what is "enough"? When your
body's demand for nutrients is satisfied?

Nonsense!

Let's face facts. We eat until we are full or until we have that
"full" feeling. When we talk about being full, we mean our
stomach is full and we feel satiated.

That's one of the major reasons why most weight-loss diets
fail. You are being told to eat less, but when you do, your
stomach is always half empty and you are constantly hungry.
That's when you decide that your diet is ridiculous and you are
not going to starve all your life, and so you blow your diet and
go back to eating as before.

If you rate your stomach as "large," there is an almost 100
percent chance that you always feel hungry when on a diet; it
is this hungry feeling that causes the constant "empty" feeling
in your stomach. "Enough is enough," you say, "I can't feel
hungry all my life."—and you quit the diet.

How often have I heard that story? Diet books and health
professionals in the weight-control field rarely tell people how
to avoid the constant feeling of being hungry. And it is so easy
to do!

ELIMINATING THE "EMPTY" FEELING

Within certain limits, our stomach can shrink and expand. Despite the fact that we can stretch the stomach by always overstuffing it with foods, this is rarely the true problem with weight control.

The real problem is in the density and content of specific foods in your diet. Or, to put it another way, we stuff ourselves with foods that induce the hunger feeling and that are low in volume and high in calories at the same time. By the time our stomach says "full," we have consumed an excess of calories. The trick now is to induce the feeling of being satieted, the feeling of being full, with fewer calories.

It can be done! We can achieve it by bringing two dietary variables, fats and fiber, to within desired ranges.

Fats, as you know, are very high in calories (9 calories per gram). In the average American diet, about 40 percent to 42 percent of all the calories are derived from fats. This, according to the experts in heart disease, cancer, and diabetes, is far too high. The opinions among the various researchers fluctuate a bit, but they will all agree that it should be somewhere from 25 percent to 34 percent.

As you have seen in chapter 3, fats serve a number of important functions in the body, from supplying essential fatty acids to serving as insulating material and padding for the organs in our body. Dr. Robert Atkins demonstrated repeatedly that a small amount of fat helps to give you the "satiated" feeling, but twice as much fat won't make you feel twice as satisfied—it will only make you look fat. Also, as we pointed out earlier, the activity of a fat-forming enzyme that makes you hungry for fat foods, increases in your body when the diet is either far too low or too high in fats. So you see that bringing the fat content of your diet to within the right range is very important.

ESTIMATING AND CALCULATING THE FATS AND FIBER IN YOUR DIET

Check Table 3.3. If you eat the all-American diet and consume some of these foods on a regular basis, the percentage of calories derived from fats will be in the 40 percent range.

If you always choose low-fat or non-fat over whole-milk products; prefer broiled or baked over fried foods; eat very little red meat; use butter or margarine sparingly; and consume good amounts of vegetables, greens, and other complex carbohydrates, your percentage of calories from fats will be in the 33 percent range. If you want it to be lower, you must be even stricter.

If you want to calculate the percentage of fats in your diet, add up all the calories you consume in a typical day. To compute the number of fat calories, add up all the grams of fats in your foods and multiply the number by nine. Then calculate the percentage of these fat calories in the total calories. If this is too complicated, don't worry: To know the exact numbers is not really important; and if you want to have your nutrition evaluated in detail, you can always use one of the computer programs recommended in the appendix.

Professor Denis Burkitt of Australia demonstrated that a high-fiber diet can almost totally eliminate cancer of the colon. To classify a diet as truly high in fiber, large amounts of vegetables, salads, whole-grain products, and fruits must be part of your daily food intake. Increasing fiber moves the food through the digestive tract faster and prevents cancer-causing chemicals from forming; it also regulates bowel movements.

A NUTRITION-COURSE LABORATORY EXPERIMENT

To demonstrate the connection between caloric intake and the amount of fats and fiber in the diet, we designed a simple experiment for our biochemistry students. They were given round glass containers approximately the size of the human stomach. We asked them to "stuff the stomachs" with one of two different types of food, which we had purchased earlier: (1) cheeseburgers, french fries, and milk shakes from a fast-food chain; or (2) broiled fish, green salad, vegetables, whole grain bread, and tea or coffee.

The caloric contents of all the foods were known to the students. When the two "stomachs" were filled to the top, the calories and nutritional quality of the two diets were compared. The difference in calories between the fast-food and the high-quality meals ranged from 500 calories to 800 calories per stomach filling. Not only did the high-quality meal have fewer calories, but it also had less fats, more fiber, and a higher vitamin and mineral content, so the students could actually see that the stomach with the high-quality food was nutritionally sounder and as physically full.

We have now demonstrated that you can feel full and satisfied by actually eating fewer calories and a better diet. Isn't that ideal and what we want? Who could ask for more?

THE REAL PROBLEM WITH FAST (OR JUNK) FOODS

Take a look at Table 4.1. Most of our fast foods are extremely low in volume and high in fats. When we are in a hurry and stop at a fast-food place, a warning signal should go off in our heads. Over the past years a few fast-food chains have tried to improve the quality of their food by giving people a choice of salads and other fresh foods. So, if you really feel that you have to eat at one of those places, and can't come up with a better choice, at least include a green salad and don't drown it in the dressing. But beware! Your chance of controlling your caloric intake by eating at fast-food places and feeling full and satisfied at the same time is extremely small. Just look at Table 4.1 and decide on the minimum amount of food you would like to eat in one day, and then add up the calories. It's almost impossible to come out ahead.

RAW VEGETABLES ARE OFTEN CALLED "NEGATIVE-CALORIE FOODS"

Since many raw vegetables contain only a small number of calories, and since the body has to expend some energy in digesting them, an overall negative calorie count would result if you would eat only these foods. A stomach filled with these

Table 4.1
Caloric Content of Fast Foods

Company	Food	Calories
Arby's	Ham and cheese	458
	Super roast beef sandwich	705
Baskin Robbins	1 scoop ice cream with sugar cone	200 (approx)
Burger Chef	Big Chef	542
	Mariner Platter	680
	Skipper's Treat	604
Burger King	Whopper	606
Dunkin Donuts	1 donut	250 (approx)
Kentucky Fried Chicken	Extra crispy dinner	950
	1 keel	283
	1 thigh	276
McDonald's	Egg McMuffin	352
	Hotcakes w/butter and syrup	472
	Big Mac	541
	French fries	211
	Quarter pounder w/cheese	518
	Apple pie	300
	Chocolate shake	364
Taco Bell	Beef Burrito	466
	Taco	186
	Beef Tostada	291

foods would contain much fewer calories than your body needs, and this is one of the reasons why these foods are called "negative-calorie foods."

A nutritional analysis of these foods would show that the majority of them are very low in protein but high in vitamins and minerals. This is the reason why they should be combined with foods from Table 3.2. You literally can eat unlimited amounts of these foods; have some of them in your refrigerator for whenever the urge to snack strikes you.

COMPUTERS PROVE OUR POINT

We wanted to find out how many calories a person could save by changing from an average American diet to one that is low in fats and high in fiber.

Using one of the computer programs designed by our research group, we did a detailed analysis of the food intake of a number of people who were consuming a typical American diet that derived 42 percent of its calories from fats and 25 percent from refined carbohydrates.

We then recalculated the diets after we substituted some of the "bad" calories (one-fourth of the fats and half of the refined carbohydrates) with vegetables, whole-grain products, and fruits. The total calories were left untouched.

What did we find? As we changed from an "average American diet" to a diet lower in fats and refined carbohydrates and higher in natural foods, the following changes were observed:

1. The volume of the foods increased by 20 percent to 30 percent while the total calories remained the same. This means that a person on the high-quality diet would get the "full" signal from the stomach when 20 percent to 30 percent fewer calories were consumed. For a person on a 2,500-calories-a-day diet, this would mean a 500-to-750-calories savings per day, accounting for a weight loss of four to seven pounds per month.

2. Vitamin intake increased by 400 percent to 700 percent. Mineral intake also increased and important mineral ratios became more normal. Fiber increased by 300 percent to 600 percent.

If these same people were to go on an additional 40-minute walk each day, the total weight loss per month would increase to 6.5 pounds to 10 pounds per month.

So you see, calorie counting *is* important, and weight loss *is* easy.

FIBER SUPPLEMENTS

A number of fiber formulations, made from apple, rice, or the Konjac root, are also available as supplements.

Glucomannan, the fiber prepared from the Konjac root, has received quite a bit of attention as a weight-loss preparation. It is a natural fiber, with no artificial additives, and comes in tablet and capsule form. It is safe when taken in the recommended amounts.

Every fiber, from rice to wheat bran, from carrot pulp to citrus roughage, absorbs water, taking up more space and filling up your stomach. Glucomannan absorbs much more water than any of these fibers.

Fiber tablets are usually taken about thirty minutes before a meal. The idea is to fill at least part of the stomach with this fiber so that people will eat less when they sit down for a meal.

A number of nutritionists like this idea, but I'd rather see people get the fiber from natural foods that also supply vitamins and minerals. Personally, I only recommend it to people who sometimes have no choice but to eat a low-fiber, high-fat meal.

We recently learned that the FDA has launched a preliminary review of the Kellogg Company advertising for its All-Bran Cereal, because the ads claim that the cereal can help to prevent cancer.

Why would our own FDA want to prevent people from getting this basic message, especially when this method of cancer-prevention is clearly supported by data published in the medical literature. If, after reading all this medical literature one still doubts that fiber can help to prevent cancer, one might as well doubt that the sun will rise the next day.

Their problem is deep-rooted. The FDA has a few extremely out-dated regulations. One of them states that if any food, or component of a food, is found to be effective in dealing with a disease, it must be classified as a drug and must be treated like one, become a prescription item, and so forth. In the light of the many recent findings that connect hundreds of foods, vitamins, or minerals, with the onset, prevention, or even treatment of specific diseases, FDA regulations like these, even in the kindest terms, must be called outright idiocy. Instead of changing their regulations, they hassle over details, and the public becomes more and more confused. If one would apply FDA regulations by the letter, carrots, bran, and the antioxidant vitamins would already have to be classified as drugs. These foods would therefore have to be locked up in a special drug section of your store, and dispensing them would require a prescription from your doctor.

Are you cracking up over so much ignorance? Read more about this in health magazines and you will be amazed to find out how many branches of the medical establishment would like to make vitamins or other foods prescription items.

A final calculation for a diet that includes glucomannan

Counting calories *can* be easy. Let's assume that you are on a 2,800-calories-a-day diet. The daily caloric intake can be lowered by 1,100 calories a day without undergoing any stress at all.

1. Use glucomannan before just two of the major meals, lunch and dinner. By filling part of the stomach with this natural fiber, food intake is reduced by at least 10 percent—a full feeling is reached earlier, and at least 200 calories a day are saved.

2. Change the overall diet to less fats, less sugar, more natural foods, and more greens. As demonstrated in our computer study, this can reduce the overall food intake by at least 500 calories a day.

3. In addition to regular physical activity, take a thirty-minute walk each day. This certainly isn't asking too much and can save another 200 calories a day.

4. Another 200 calories a day can be saved by not eating one candy bar, not drinking one beer or cola, or not eating any other unneeded food.

If you add up all the calories in steps 1-4, multiply the number by 7, and then divide by 3,500, you get 2.3 pounds saved per week; about 10 pounds saved per month.

Try to think of other ways to save or burn a few more calories per day. Counting calories, especially if these are easy calories, works.

Since sufficient fiber is an important factor in preventing digestive tract cancer, in eliminating some heart disease risk factors, and in increasing the oxygen supply to the tissues (via reducing the percentage of fat in the diet), it is also a definite anti-aging factor.

ADDITIONAL WAYS TO REDUCE OR ELIMINATE HUNGER FEELINGS

If, after following our advice, you are still bothered by persistant hunger feelings, after or in-between meals, try any one of the following three hunger-reduction methods. These methods are not perfect, but research data and good responses from our weight-loss candidates warrant telling you about them.

The first two methods involve pressure points, and Dr. Richard Passwater, in *The Easy No-Flab Diet*, described them as follows:

Method 1:

Insert your index fingers gently into your ears with the palms turned toward your face. Place your thumbs on the tragus, the little bump of cartilage at the front of your external ear. Firmly massage the tragus between your thumbs and index fingers for at least one minute.

Method 2:

Place your index fingers in the small depressions immediately in front of your ears, just slightly higher than the tragus. Rub in a circular motion for at least one minute.

Method 3:

The third method is based on behavioral research by Johns Hopkins University researchers. Dr. Maria Simonson found that staring at a piece of pink paper (the exact name of the color is Baker-Miller pink) will send a message to the brain that has a calming effect and that takes the edge off your hunger. So, the next time you get that urge to snack between meals, try one of these methods. It certainly won't hurt you.

There are a number of natural methods of appetite-control

that utilize pills that contain different amino acid combinations. Even though there might be a scientific basis for some of them, we have found that in all our weight-loss patients who tried these pills, the results were negative.

NOW GO TO FIGURE 10.1 AND CHECK ITEM 4

You should now know that there is a relation between the consumption of fats and of fiber and weight loss. Estimate if, and to what degree, you should lower the fat content and increase the fiber in your diet.

    4.a. Further reduce fats.
    4.b. Further increase fiber.

5

WEIGHT IS WHEN YOU EAT—The wrong eating patterns can amount to 30 pounds per year.

> I once counseled a woman who merely had to quit her late night snack and eat some breakfast in order to shed the desired weight.
>
> Richard Passwater, Ph.D.
> Author of *The Easy No-Flab Diet*

CHECK YOURSELF

"Eat a regular breakfast, don't skip meals, and don't eat rich late-night snacks," is basic advice we often hear in a nutrition course. Only very recently nutrition research demonstrated that skipping meals and irregular eating patterns is associated with a weight gain, instead of a weight loss. Understanding body chemistry allows us to interpret these findings.

1. Do you always eat a good breakfast? YES NO
2. Do you eat regular meals? YES NO
3. Do you make an effort to have your dinner early in the evening, before 7 P.M.? YES NO
4. Do you often have late-night snacks? YES NO

If you answered "YES" to the first three questions and "NO" to item 4, you can skip this chapter, check "Already doing" for item 5 in Figure 10.1, and move on to the next chapter.

When I directed a weight-loss study at a local college and evaluated the health practices of the participants, we were surprised to learn that more than 95 percent of the weight-loss candidates had given negative answers for the two key questions:

Do you eat a regular breakfast?

Do you eat dinner before 7 P.M.?

This brought back some memories from a physiology class I once took at the University of Munich Medical School. The lecturer had been involved in weight-loss studies and found that faulty eating patterns were a major cause of weight gain.

In later years, many other research groups emphasized these findings, and it was always suggested that irregular eating patterns caused a person to eat more. Yet, many people are convinced that they will lose weight by skipping meals.

IT'S *WHEN* YOU EAT THAT MATTERS

Two studies, one conducted in England, and the other here in the United States, finally answered all our questions. In a study headed by Dr. James Marston, a group of overweight people was literally locked up in a building. Divided into two groups, they all received the same type of foods and the same number of calories. One group ate an early breakfast, a small lunch, and an even smaller dinner. The other group consisted of people who refused to eat breakfast, had lunch, then had a larger dinner. After about ten weeks, the early breakfast eaters had lost an average of 14 pounds, whereas the late eaters had lost only about 12 pounds. This clearly demonstrated that foods eaten early in the day have less of a chance of being deposited as fat than foods eaten later in the day.

In the United States, Dr. R. Graeber of the Walter Reed Medical Center conducted a similar study and found that less weight is gained per calorie when food is consumed in the earlier part of the day instead of in the afternoon or evening.

Other weight-control experts who noted what people were eating while on their usual diets, when they were gaining weight, suggested that the difference in weight loss between the two eating patterns can be as much as one pound per week. This again confirms the importance of eating a good, balanced breakfast.

People who want to lose weight often believe that they can save calories by not eating breakfast. *Not so!* Skipping breakfast makes you hungrier, and in many cases, people eat more during the remaining two meals, with the extra calories deposited as fat.

A Look at What Is Going On Inside the Body

It is a well-established fact that it is easier to deposit fat in your body than to burn it up. Why is this so? Can we explain these findings?

Our body stores energy mainly in two forms: (1) as fat in the adipose tissue, and (2) as glycogen in the liver and lean muscle mass.

Glycogen consists of long chains of glucose hooked together. When the blood-sugar (glucose) level falls below a normal range, glycogen is taken apart and glucose is released back into the blood, thus, keeping the blood-sugar level within a normal range.

In the morning, blood-sugar levels are usually on the low side, and the storage places for glucose, the liver and the lean muscle mass, are low on glycogen.

Morning is also the time when most people begin their day and when they start burning calories. Since our body has a priority to keep the blood sugar within normal ranges, if we don't eat breakfast, the body must find other ways to add glucose to the bloodstream. Pathways to utilize fat deposits in order to keep the blood-sugar level normal are extremely limited, and there is only the muscle mass as a reserve.

When the body has a need to increase the blood-sugar level, and all other reserves are exhausted, the following *undesirable* emergency reaction occurs: Lean muscle mass is broken down into its building blocks, the amino acids; then, the amino acids are converted to glucose. We therefore lose the desirable lean muscle mass instead of unwanted fat. Since most calorie-burning reactions take place in the lean muscle mass, a reduced, lean muscle mass also means a reduced metabolism, and weight loss becomes even more difficult.

Why does a big meal at night make us grow fat (and feel tired)?

During the night hours and when we sleep, we slow down our activity, and our metabolism is at its lowest point; therefore, the carbohydrates that wind up in the body as glucose are stored as glycogen, and any excess is converted into fat. Since the large muscles are not being used to do work, the burning of fat has also been reduced to a minimum, and more fat now appears in the bloodstream. We say that the level of triglycerides (the fats in the blood) is high. Examination of the blood after a meal high in fats shows that blood cells clot together in rows of five to ten blood cells. Since the capillaries through which the blood supplies the various organs with oxygen are very narrow, and even single cells often have to twist to make it through, the oxygen supply to the organs is greatly reduced. It is this reduced oxygen supply that makes you feel tired.

When fat is not burned, it is stored in the adipose tissue. Extra glucose, from a big dinner or from a late-night snack that is not burned or stored, is also converted into fat.

Your Shape Also Goes Down the Drain

When you exercise in the morning, without first eating a good breakfast, you also force your body to do some strange things.

In the morning, blood sugar levels are on the low side. When you start exercising you use up this fuel and levels drop even further. A top priority of your body is to maintain blood sugar levels within normal ranges. Glycogen storage in the liver and muscle mass is quickly depleted, and your body now uses an emergency reaction to maintain a reasonable blood sugar level. It takes muscle mass apart into the building blocks, the amino acids, and then it changes the amino acids to glucose. The end-result is a muscle loss.

We recently checked this concept in women who had difficulty rebuilding muscle mass even though they exercised; upon closer examination, we found that not one of them ate a good breakfast. When they started to eat at least some protein and carbohydrates for breakfast, before they exercised, rebuilding muscle mass became much easier. (Note: after eating breakfast, wait about fifteen to thirty minutes before you begin to exercise.)

Remember, muscle consists of protein, and you have to supply it with protein in order to build muscle. You wouldn't expect a builder to construct a house for you without building materials, would you?

If You Can't Eat Breakfast, Drink It!

We are creatures of habit.

"NO, I just can't eat breakfast, and I won't!" We hear this quite often from people who come to our office and who want a magic pill that is supposed to make them lose weight and look better without any effort on their part.

We have a better solution for those of you who don't want to eat any breakfast and for others who don't have the time. Would it be asking too much of you to go to the refrigerator and drink half a glass of a prepared breakfast drink? Certainly not! Anybody can do that!

All that you have to do at night, before you go to bed, is prepare a breakfast drink. You can mix all kinds of goodies in it; anything you like, as long as it contains some protein, none or *very little* sugar, and maybe some fruit. The basic ingredients should be yogurt, kefir, low- or nonfat milk, and protein powder. Mix these basic ingredients in any proportion that you find appealing, with or without fruit.

Since your body also needs roughage, eat an apple or some other fruit while on your way to work or just chew on a few bran tablets. Bran is an excellent source of roughage, and you might include a small amount of it in your drink.

Now you have protein, some carbohydrates, a small amount of fat, and some roughage. This drink also allows you to wash down some of the vitamins you need. Is this asking too much from you? For your health?

FASTING OR STARVATION

A number of good things have been reported about fasting. Underfeeding and fasting in animals has increased life spans dramatically. It can also be helpful in cleansing the body of toxic substances and in determining special allergies. However, when it comes to weight loss, we feel that it can do more harm than good because rebuilding lean muscle mass becomes impossible, and muscle loss is a definite risk. As observed in our own group, and also reported elsewhere, most overweight people have far below acceptable amounts of lean muscle mass on their bodies, and rebuilding it becomes a top priority.

"Why not?" asked a friend. "If I don't eat anything, I'll save all those calories and lose the weight much faster."

Not so! Take a look at Figure 5.1.

When you fast (no caloric intake, just water), energy is taken from your fat and your muscle mass. You can afford to lose the fat but not the muscle mass. The following two major processes take place in your body: Fat from the adipose tissue is mobilized and goes into the Krebs (energy) cycle. However, when you fast, there are no carbohydrates to go into the Krebs cycle—a requirement for the big incinerator to burn efficiently—therefore, the fats are burned inefficiently and wind up as ketones. Ketones change the pH of your body, increase urination, wash minerals out of your body, and do a lot of other bad things to your body. These are the symptoms of diabetes, and the general condition is known as "ketosis." Muscle mass is also lost because the body breaks it down to get amino acids, which, in turn, are changed to glucose to maintain the blood-sugar level within reasonable ranges. Since very little of this glucose can go into the Krebs cycle, it therefore burns inefficiently, and the muscle loss causes a decrease in your metabolism.

Did you see the movie *Gandhi*? When Gandhi went on a hunger strike and was starving himself, his body soon looked like a skeleton with skin stretched over it. Not eating breakfast or exercising on an empty stomach are two milder forms of starvation. The loss of muscle mass is a great risk, and even

Figure 5.1. Fasting or Starvation—merely a stricter form of not eating breakfast or exercising on an empty stomach.

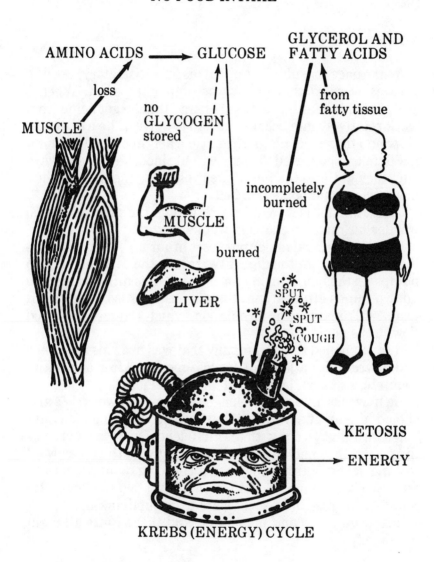

NO FOOD INTAKE

AMINO ACIDS ⟶ GLUCOSE

GLYCEROL AND FATTY ACIDS

loss

MUSCLE

no GLYCOGEN stored

from fatty tissue

MUSCLE

incompletely burned

LIVER

burned

SPUT
SPUT
COUGH

KETOSIS

ENERGY

KREBS (ENERGY) CYCLE

if you exercise, a gain in muscle mass is very unlikely under these conditions.

A CASE HISTORY

A man once consulted me about his (unsatisfactory) sex life. He was worried that he was becoming impotent. When I evaluated his health practices, I found that he got home from work relatively late because he had to drive quite a distance. He would then meet his girlfriend at a neighborhood bar for a few drinks. They loved the movies, but since they were always late, they got into the habit of eating after the movie. Then more drinks and home into bed.

On a full stomach, with no rest, plus the alcohol, it's no wonder his male mechanism wouldn't work.

Blood has several major purposes in our body. It transports the nutrients from the digestive tract to the cells, and it also pumps up the penis during an erection. It is difficult for it to do two things efficiently at the same time! Also, overweight people often have poor circulation, which reduces the blood flow to the penis.

It so happened that a company that was near his residence had offered him a job, but for less money. After our initial counseling session, he decided to take the job.

He now was able to sleep longer and walk to work. We also signed him up at a health club where he worked out on days when he didn't go out with his girlfriend. On days when they did go out, they had an early dinner first, and then they went to a movie. Sometimes they had a relaxing drink with their friends after the movie, but his girlfriend told me later: "He now feels so good, he doesn't want to go out drinking, he just wants to go home and make love; and that's quite all right with me."

NOW GO TO FIGURE 10.1 AND CHECK ITEM 5

Item #5 deals with regular food intake. This either applies to you or it doesn't. How strict you are with yourself depends very much on how many changes you are willing to make, and how fast you want to achieve results. At least make some changes toward more regular eating patterns and see how it works. When you recognize how well this works for your weight loss, you will probably be more willing to tighten the reins.

6

VITAMINS AND MINERALS: The magic bullets in the fight against diseases and aging.

> Television host, talking to Richard Simmons: "There was a time when you were obese. What made you lose the weight? We see so many people going on a weight-loss program and losing a few pounds, and then they quit their diet. What kept you going?"
>
> Richard Simmons: "I just didn't want to die!"
>
> Channel 11, TV
> Los Angeles
> November 18, 1983

CHECK YOURSELF

Vitamins and minerals. Are you confused? In this chapter we explain why taking supplements is especially important when on a weight-loss program and why health experts in preventive medicine feel that the RDA (Recommended Daily Allowance) for vitamins is insufficient to achieve the best possible health. We also point out the medical publications that demonstrated a lack of certain vitamins as heart disease and cancer risk factors, and why a group of vitamins and minerals were so effective in interfering with the true causes of aging.

1. Do you have a supplementation program that is based on a nutrition professional's advice?   YES   NO
2. Do you always take your supplements with food?   YES   NO
3. Do you take a multivitamin with minerals?   YES   NO
4. Do you take some extra Vitamin C with flavonoids?   YES   NO
5. If you take selenium and Vitamin E, do you take them together, at night, and not in combination with Vitamin C?   YES   NO

If you answered "YES" to all five questions, you can skip this chapter and check "Already doing" for item 6 in Figure 10.1.

But since there is so much confusion about this topic, why don't you read it anyway or possibly come back to it later.

VITAMINS

While the Federal Drug Administration (FDA) tells us that the RDA of vitamins is sufficient for good health, numerous publications in preventive medicine suggest that four to six times the RDA should be the minimum recommended level for optimum health. Even the most conservative researchers in the vitamin field agree that a supplement of about two times the RDA of the fat soluble vitamins (A, D, E, and K) and about five to ten times the RDA of the water soluble vitamins (B complex and C) has absolutely no chance of doing any harm.

Some of the most convincing data that suggest a much larger need for vitamins in humans have been published by Professor E. Cheraskin of the University of Alabama, School of Medicine.

Professor Cheraskin uses computer techniques to check the

intake of specific vitamins as he moves from a sample of the "average" population (those who have a number of minor medical complaints) to a group of people who are perfectly healthy and have no medical complaints. He has done this so far for vitamin C, niacin, and vitamin A, and each time he finds that the vitamin intake increases from slightly below the RDA level for the average person to four to six times the RDA level for the healthy subjects.

MINERALS

The RDAs are more reasonable for minerals, but as many computer evaluations of the average American diet have shown, most people are far below the RDA in their mineral intake. For selenium, for example, a very important mineral in respect to cancer prevention, the average diet contains about 100 to 150 micrograms per day. According to Professor G. Schrauzer, of the University of Southern California at San Diego, optimum cancer protection is achieved at a level of about 300 micrograms per day.

Simple imbalances of minerals in the diet (i.e., not enough calcium, and too much phosphorous) can induce disorders such as secondary hyperparathyroidism (an overactive thyroid). Minerals have not shared the same spotlight as vitamins; they tend to be forgotten. When you take your vitamins, be sure they are supported by all the minerals.

AN UPDATE ON THE LATEST VITAMIN AND MINERAL RESEARCH

Are you confused? Don't know whether or not to take vitamins and minerals? Since there is so much misinformation and scientific dishonesty concerning vitamins and minerals, by taking a look at some of the key data in this field, you can decide for yourself if you want to take supplements. To make it easier for you, we'll even give you a choice of two supplementation programs: one more conservative, the other more aggressive.

What we generally hear about vitamins is a cross section of facts, fallacies, opinions, and ignorance, with many members of the orthodox medical profession set against vitamins. One often gets the impression that the medical profession is afraid of Mother Nature's little helpers. Are they worried that the vitamin store might replace the drug store?

Let's look at some basic facts. At first, there was the minimum daily requirement (MDR). Minimum daily requirement for what? To keep you from dropping dead right now? Certainly not for optimum health. Later, it was demonstrated in a number of scientific publications that the MDR definitely was *not* sufficient for a large number of people. So, they raised the MDR by 50 percent and called it the RDA.

Then, there were two sets of publications concerning vitamins and minerals. The first demonstrated that the average person doesn't get the RDA of vitamins from food alone. Similar literature also showed that the mineral intake for most people was below the RDA (Table 6.1). In one of our own research projects, we determined the vitamin and mineral intake of people who came to see their doctor because "they didn't feel well" and compared it to a number of healthy people who followed good nutrition and other health practices. Even though the healthy control group had a slightly higher vitamin and mineral intake, neither group received their RDA or more from food sources alone (Table 6.2).

The second set of publications demonstrated that the vitamin intake for optimum functioning (lowest risk, maximum disease prevention) is anywhere from four to eight times the RDA. RDAs for many minerals were not established or were not taken by the average population. The data come from longevity studies on animals and nutrition evaluations on humans, (utilizing the Cornell Medical Index Questionnaire). (See Figure 6.1.)

These are just a few studies that should have made the headlines in health-related publications. I have talked to numerous anti-vitamin doctors during medical meetings, and none of them had ever heard of these important and up-to-date publications. One major responsibility of a scientist is to

Table 6.1
Problems with the Average American Diet

Number of nutrients	Number of subjects	Percentage of subjects*
1	873	5.8
2	931	6.2
3	962	6.4
4	1003	6.7
5	1018	6.8
6	1008	6.7
7	944	6.3
8	852	5.7
9	798	5.3
10	763	5.1
11	815	5.4
12	706	4.7
13	607	4.0
14	464	3.1
15	352	2.3
16	325	2.2
17	253	1.7
Total		84.4

Source: E. Cheraskin, M.D., University of Alabama, School of Medicine (Dec. 1976). Meeting of the International Academy of Preventive Medicine, Spring 1977.

*Percentage of 15,050 subjects not meeting the RDA for 1 to 17 nutrients as determined from a food-frequency questionnaire data bank.

Table 6.2
Vitamin and Mineral Intake of Patients
Versus Health Controls

The premise that if you eat a cross section of different foods, your body gets all the vitamins and minerals it needs is not correct.

Vitamin and Mineral Intake

The standard employed, even though we feel it is an irrational one, was the RDA. Our findings demonstrate that even healthy people, with good eating habits, don't always get the RDA of all vitamins. Furthermore, Cheraskin and Ringsdorf (1976) presented data showing that the ideal intake of niacin and vitamin A is from five to eight times the RDA.

	Percentage of people who received, from food sources alone, 100% or more of the RDA of:		
	All 11 vitamins[a]	Any 8 of 11 vitamins	Any 6 of 11 vitamins
Patients	2%	20%	48%
Healthy controls	44%	100%	100%
	Percentage of people who received, from food sources alone, 100% or more of the RDA of:		
	All 8 minerals[b]	Any 5 of 8 minerals	Any 4 of 8 minerals
Patients	0%	16%	26%
Healthy controls	18%	92%	100%

[a]The 11 vitamins checked were: A, E, C, B1, B2, B3, B6, B12, folic acid, pantothenic acid, and biotin.
[b]The 8 minerals checked were: calcium, phosphorus, magnesium, iron, copper, zinc, iodine, and manganese.

Source: Kugler, Hans J., *Journal of the International Academy of Preventive Medicine* (Winter 1977): 79-85.

Figure 6.1. The Cheraskin Model for Higher Human Vitamin Needs (utilizing the Cornell Medical Index Questionnaire).

Number of subjects in study: 1,500
Average medical complaints per month: 15
Procedure: Reduce the number of complaints, one by one, to zero and follow: (1) niacin and (2) vitamin A intake.
Summary of findings: As we move from the sample group of 1,500 (average 15 medical complaints, slightly below the RDA for vitamins) to the smaller group with no complaints (best possible state of health), the average intake of both vitamins goes to about four to eight times the RDA.

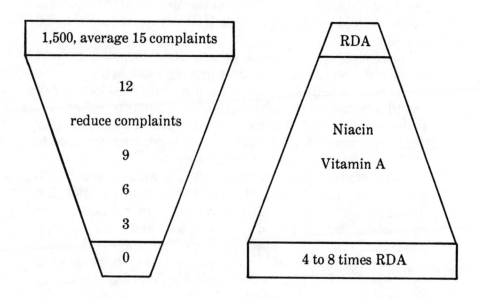

Note: From E. Cheraskin, M.D., *Intl. J. Vit. & Nutr. Res.* Volume 46 (Dec. 1976).

be up-to-date in what is being published in the literature. Obviously, far too many health professionals are too busy making money instead of reading the literature.

Many of the latest findings about vitamins were presented in my book *Dr. Kugler's Seven Keys to a Longer Life*. Other excellent books are *Supernutrition* and *Supernutrition for Healthy Hearts* by Dr. Richard Passwater, and *Meganutrition* by Dr. Richard Kunin. Also see *The Vitamin C Connection*, by E. Cheraskin, M.D.

High-density and low-density lipoproteins (HDL and LDL) are two cholesterol-carrying fractions in the blood. The HDL level is low in many people. High levels of HDL have been associated with a lower heart disease risk. After supplementing patients' diets with 600 milligrams of vitamin E per day for one month, Dr. W. Herman, of the Memorial City General Hospital in Houston, found that HDL levels increased by 50 percent.

Nutritional supplements greatly increased the IQ and many physical functions of the mentally retarded.

Higher concentrations of vitamin A in the blood serve as a shield against cancer. Researchers at Radcliffe Infirmary, Oxford, England, examined blood samples of 16,000 men for vitamin A content. Higher vitamin A levels corresponded to lower incidences of various types of cancer.

The average American gets about 100 micrograms to 150 micrograms of selenium (a trace mineral) in the diet. Reduced rates of many types of cancer, including breast cancer in women, were observed in people who had a higher selenium intake. Animal experiments confirmed these findings.

Longevity studies and immunologic research, performed by Professor Roy Walford of UCLA's School of Medicine, demonstrated that increases in the life span of animals can be achieved with antioxidant (vitamins C, E, A, and the trace mineral selenium) supplementation.

Even the *Journal of the American Medical Association* (JAMA) is now reporting good findings about supplements. One of the articles reported that in a group of fifty-seven healthy young men and women (ages ranged from 18 to 35), the ones who took one gram of calcium supplement per day for twenty weeks had a significant reduction in blood pressure.

NOW GO TO FIGURE 10.1 and CHECK ITEM 6

Before you decide if you want to take supplements and at what level to start, be sure you understand the reasons for taking vitamins and minerals.

When going on a weight-loss program, your food intake is reduced, and therefore, your intake of vitamins and minerals is also reduced. The program also induces a certain degree of stress because of some of the changes you will make. Both of these conditions are helped by taking supplements. In addition, some of the vitamins and minerals will also help to prevent diseases and interfere with the true causes of aging. Vitamins and minerals do not cause you to lose weight; they are taken as health insurance.

This need for supplementation during weight-loss was confirmed in a study by Dr. A. Belko and his colleagues, who found that women's riboflavin requirements increase when on a weight-loss program that restricted calories and included exercise.

Depending on how willing you are to take supplements, and how perfect you want to be in achieving your best possible health, we would like to give you a choice of a conservative supplementation program and an aggressive supplementation program. The following list will help you get started.

1. *A conservative but reasonably sufficient program*
   Always with food (breakfast or lunch):
   1 multivitamin with minerals
   2 additional multimineral tablets (they all come in approximately the same size)
   1 vitamin C with flavonoids (500 mg)
2. *The aggressive program*
   With breakfast:
   1 multivitamin with minerals
   2 additional multimineral tablets
   1 vitamin C with flavonoids (500 mg)

10,000 to 25,000 I.U. of vitamin A
With lunch or around midday:
1 B complex (25 mg to 50 mg range)
1 vitamin C with flavonoids (500 mg)
After dinner or at bedtime
200 to 400 I.U. of vitamin E
100 to 150 mcg (micrograms) of selenium (yeast based).
1 calcium-magnesium or multimineral tablet.

Special supplements to increase endurance and stamina will be discussed in chapter 7.

For other supplements interfering with aging, such as sulfur amino acids, BHT, procaine, etc., see chapter 16. A more detailed approach to supplementation and dealing with allergies is outlined in *The Supernutrition Handbook* by P. Mooney. This book is not available in bookstores; see the bibliography for information on how to get it. (Note: Always discuss your supplementation program with your doctor, who will hopefully be nutrition oriented.) Write to IAHHM for a list of nutrition- and prevention-oriented doctors in your area.

If you already have your own supplemental program, check "Already doing" for item #6 in Figure 10.1.

7

FACTOR #7
PHYSICAL ACTIVITY: From the treatment of depression to sexercise.

> A rolling stone gathers no fat.
> Wayne Spence, M.D.

Figure 7.1. Do You Suffer from Depression?

TAKE THIS TEST NOW.

The following is a list of symptoms or feelings people sometimes have. Read each statement and then, according to your own definition, check off how often you had these symptoms or feelings during the past week. Circle only one number for each statement. The ratings are as follows:

    0 means you never have the symptom or feeling.
    1 means it is mild when it occurs or it occurs only occasionally.
    2 means moderate or occurring at least once per week.
    3 means severe, or occuring frequently.

1) More negative than positive thoughts	0 1 2 3
2) Decreased energy, no "umph"	0 1 2 3
3) Feeling depressed	0 1 2 3
4) Worrying excessively	0 1 2 3

5) Reduced sex drive	0	1	2	3
6) Loss of sexual pleasure	0	1	2	3
7) Suicidal thoughts or tendencies	0	1	2	3
8) Feeling trapped in a situation	0	1	2	3
9) Just sitting there, brooding over things	0	1	2	3
10) Feeling insecure or low self-esteem	0	1	2	3
11) Feeling lonely; nobody needs you	0	1	2	3
12) Tears flow easily	0	1	2	3
13) You feel that everything is an effort	0	1	2	3

Your tentative depression score: add up all numbers: _____

CHECK YOURSELF

Do you have any physical-activity program that fulfills the following minimum requirements:

1. Does it have a warm-up before and a cool-down after the activity? YES NO

2. Is it done at least three times per week? YES NO

3. Is it performed, uninterrupted, for at least 30 minutes to 40 minutes each time? YES NO

4. Is it vigorous, with your pulse rate
   in the right range?   YES   NO

5. Is your score less than 10 points on
   the depression chart? (See Fig.
   7.1.)   YES   NO

If you answered "YES" to all five questions, you can skip this chapter, check "Already doing" for item 7 in Figure 10.1, and move on to the next chapter.

A lack of exercise is a risk factor for heart disease, diabetes, depression, arthritis, and eating disorders such as bulimia and binging; applying exercise correctly has been very helpful in treating these disorders. Weight loss without a minimum amount of physical activity is impossible.

Any physical activity is an excellent way to burn up calories; however, *you* might not have to, nor want to, do more than what you are already doing. To just burn up a few more calories, you can just increase one or more physical activities —from just parking your car a few yards farther away from the shopping mall to going for a walk with friends or by doing anything instead of just sitting.

Another way is to do the minimum amount of exercise that is required to maintain good health. This, I feel, is a very important area. Many people tell me that they're really not very excited about exercising but realize that it is important if they are to prevent heart attacks and other disorders. They want me to tell them what is the minimum exercise they should do to maintain their good health.

In this chapter and in other parts of this book, we'll give answers to "what is the minimum" questions.

HOW MUCH PHYSICAL ACTIVITY?

In England, Professor J. N. Morris has an ongoing study involving more than 30,000 government employees. He concentrates on the minimum amount of exercise every person should be doing for best possible health. In a large computer program, every person is characterized by at least thirty variables. When a person has a heart attack, the computer matches this person with others who have the same characteristics and the computer is asked, "Why did this person have a heart attack, and why didn't the others?" And each time the computer finds that the people with the lowest heart disease risk do a minimum of exercise, which is:

1. Done at least three times per week.

2. Done at least 30 minutes each time without interruptions.

3. Vigorous.

Other areas of medical research, as for example, in the treatment of diabetes and depression, confirm these minimum recommendations. So, as long as you fulfill these three minimum requirements, you can choose any exercise you like.

The emphasis in many of Professor Morris's papers is on "30 minutes as a minimum." If one does less than 30 minutes of exercise, it appears to only activate the carbohydrate metabolism without really burning fat. During the first 10 minutes to 20 minutes of exercise, the body runs mainly on the glycogen reserves. Then the fat metabolism starts to come in and fats are burned off efficiently at the 25-minute to 30-minute mark.

For people who are not used to doing exercises, walking is an excellent starting point.

HOW DO WE DEFINE "VIGOROUS?"

"Vigorous" means that your pulse (heart rate) should be in the correct range. Your maximum exercising heart rate, which should never be exceeded, is 220 minus your age. To make sure that we are always in a safe range that also gives good results, we exercise at 70 percent to 80 percent of the maximum heart rate. For a 30-year-old, the pulse rate should therefore be between 133 and 152. Several preventive medical treatments of major disorders confirm these recommendations.

Heart disease

The treatment of patients who had heart attacks, and who are now exercising to prevent another heart attack, includes exercise done at the minimum level recommended by Professor Morris. The reversal of atherosclerosis, demonstrated with angiograms (X rays of the arteries), confirms that patients are on the right track.

Diabetes

At the VA Hospital in Lexington, Kentucky, Dr. James Anderson treats adult onset diabetics with a regimen of exercise and a high-complex-carbohydrate diet.

Again, minimum amounts of exercise conform very much

to the Morris recommendations; three times per week minimum, vigorous, and a minimum of 30 minutes each time. In
some cases, the activity is a little bit less vigorous, but it is
done a little bit longer than 30 minutes.

Depression

At the University of Wisconsin, School of Medicine, Dr.
John Greist treats people who suffer from depression with a
good exercise program.

Dr. Greist is a runner himself, but he always emphasizes
that he wants his patients to exercise at least three times per
week (no matter what exercise they do), to exert themselves a
little bit (depending on their physical capacity to do exercise),
and to exercise at least for thirty to forty minutes.

His results are absolutely fantastic. Depression disappears
within two to three weeks.

Are you depressed? Figure 7.1 lists a few key questions that
deal with depression. They are usually included in tests that
have many more questions than the ones listed here, so this is
not a very precise method. Using only these questions, the
majority of people obtain scores of about 4 to 6. In cases in
which depression is suspected, scores reach 12 points to 14
points, or more. If you score in this higher range, you might
want to follow up by talking to a health professional.

Depression and Weight loss: It is extremely difficult to
motivate a person who is seriously depressed; they just sit
there, don't do anything, complain, and then they drop out. If
your depression score is high, you have already taken the most
important step to lower it; by reading this book up to this
point, you have recognized the need for a change and demonstrated the desire to make a change. You might think,
"Sounds good, but it probably won't work for me. I am
depressed for other reasons. Why should nutrition and exercise help me? They don't do anything about the actual causes
of my depression."

I could now quote hundreds of scientific papers that demonstrate the relationship between dozens of causes of depression and why nutrition and exercise are effective in solving

these problems, but I doubt that this would really convince you.

How about facing reality? You can either continue in your present state of depression, or you can take action. Since you are reading this book, I believe that you are ready to take that action and make a change.

I'll make it even easier for you so that you don't have to waste your valuable time on something about which you may not be convinced. Follow my instructions for three weeks, and I'll guarantee you that you will see dramatic, positive changes.

BULIMIA

In our counseling of bulimics, we found that the best results are achieved when vigorous exercise is done at least three to four times per week, at least forty minutes each time without interruptions, and combined with exercise machines to build lean muscle mass.

The exercise is more effective if it is combined with high-protein, low-sugar nutrition and with regular meal patterns. It is extremely important for bulimics to realize that strong exercise programs on an empty stomach (to save calories) are highly detrimental to their recovery. More in Chapter 13.

EXERCISE CALORIES AND WEIGHT LOSS

Assuming that you are presently neither gaining nor losing weight, any increase in exercise will cause a weight loss, and any decrease will cause a weight gain as shown in Figure 7.2. (Table 7.1 lists the calories burned per thirty minute exercise period.)

For example, whatever your present DCML is, if you burn an extra 500 calories per day by exercising, this amounts to one pound of weight loss per week (500 times 7, divided by 3,500). Naturally, exercising twice as much will increase the weight loss to two pounds per week.

If you take the time to study Table 7.1, you will **recognize**

Figure 7.2. The Connection Between Weight and Energy Output.

Effect of calories burned:
1. If you increase the physical activity without eating more, a weight loss will result.
2. If you decrease physical activity without eating more, a weight gain will result.

PHYSICAL ACTIVITY
(with everything else
remaining the same):

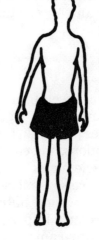

If physical activity is increased

DCML

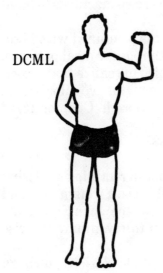

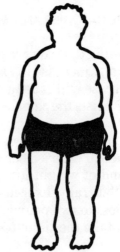

If physical activity is decreased

TABLE 7.1
Calories Burned per 30-Minute Activity Period, According to Body Weight (in pounds)

	110 lb	*150 lb*	*190 lb*
Basketball	200	280	350
Circuit training	280	380	480
Climbing hills	180	250	310
Cycling: Leisure	180	240	300
Dancing	160	210	270
Football	200	270	350
Gardening	170	230	290
Golf	130	170	210
Jazznastics	170	230	290
Judo-Karate	290	400	500
Running 8 min/mile	320	430	530
Jogging 11 min/mile	210	280	350
Skiing: Leisure	190	250	310
Hard	380	500	620
Squash	320	430	550
Swimming: Leisure	180	250	310
Hard	250	350	430
Tennis	170	220	280
Volleyball	90	110	140
Walking: Leisure	120	160	200
Hard	180	240	300

that there is a limit to weight-loss through exercise—your available time and your body's capacity to exercise are limited. You also don't want to exhaust yourself so much with exercise that you are worthless for other, more pleasurable, physical activities. (I once knew a couple in which the wife asked for a divorce because her husband always came home totally pooped from hours of playing ball.) So let's be reasonable about this.

A reasonable amount of exercise is just a little bit more than recommended earlier (three times per week, forty minutes or more, and vigorous). Go on an additipnal long walk a few times per week and you will burn the equivalent of one pound of fat in exercise calories per week. If possible, use exercise machines to build lean muscle mass. Because you are building lean muscle mass, your overall metabolism will also increase, and you'll burn an additional number of calories. Exercising not less than every second day also increases your base metabolism, which, again, helps you burn more calories.

A weight loss of one to one-and-a-half pounds per week, through caloric reductions, is reasonable and achievable. The same is true for weight loss through exercise. Together this equals two to three pounds per week; and there are many more weight-loss factors that can be applied. Weight loss can be easy if you use your common sense and learn how to do it.

INTERESTED IN SUPPLEMENTS THAT INCREASE YOUR STAMINA AND ENDURANCE?

What if you could increase your stamina with a pill; activate your body's energy reserves with a simple food extract; make exercising easier for yourself; outperform your competition at sports; be the last one to get tired at a late party? All without drugs or steroids! Nothing dangerous! Just simple food components! Impossible? Sounds too good? Not so!

Improvements in your overall nutrition and vitamin supplements will definitely increase your stamina and endurance, but there are a number of special supplements that have been utilized by athletes all over the world that can do exactly what we mentioned above. The following special supplements can be used separately or in combination, on a regular basis or only on days when you exercise or need an extra boost.

Supplements Available in the United States
Dimethyl glycine (DMG): This is a natural supplement, part of the normal human metabolism. It has been shown to increase immune functions, and it can activate high-energy phosphates that give you energy when you perform physical

tasks such as exercise. In my opinion, the best DMG is made by DaVinci or Food Science Laboratories. Take 50 milligrams to 100 milligrams of DMG per day, or slightly more if you are a very large and/or physically active person.

Liver extracts and concentrates: Generally known as "liver glandulars," these are standard supplements for improving endurance and are different from regular liver tablets. Beef liver is extracted to remove fats and other unimportant molecules. The remains are freeze-dried and pressed into tablet form. Four to six tablets per day give good results; you can take twice as much if you wish. Two good manufacturers of liver glandulars are Nutri-Dyn and Standard Process Laboratories.

Octocasonal: This extract from wheat-germ oil, was first used by the famous exercise physiologist Professor Thomas Cureton when training swimmers. Today this supplement is used in almost every sport, from football to marathon running. Take three to six minims (a measure of weight) per day, depending on the activity.

Supplements Available in Europe

Developed in West Germany, many European athletes and Olympic teams are using two natural compounds that are believed to help in building lean muscle mass and increasing endurance.

Xobaline: This is a coenzyme for vitamin B_{12}, and therefore, they are taken together. Xobaline helps in protein synthesis and, therefore, has an anabolic (muscle-building) effect. All capsules come in the 1 milligram size. One capsule per day is sufficient for most people. If you are into body building, three capsules per day are believed to give the best possible results.

Inosin: This compound is found in transfer-RNA molecules. It helps in building lean muscle mass and, therefore, also has an anabolic effect. One tablet contains 250 milligrams of inosin. A number of athletes, including myself, feel that it works best if taken about one hour before exercise. Once warmed up, one feels as if one can push weights forever.

A number of U.S. companies are hoping to make these products available in the United States, and perhaps, by the time this book is in your hands, they will be available in your health-food store or pharmacy.

SEXERCISE AND WEIGHT LOSS

Some people who believe more in positive thinking than in scientific facts might tell you that sex is the ideal exercise to lose weight and get into shape. That's not quite true. If you try to shed weight with sexercise, you might need a little help from your doctor because overweight men often have lower concentrations of sex hormones. Also, in the medical literature that deals with sex, it is generally accepted that you should get in shape to be active and good at sex, instead of the other way around.

However, sex is definitely a good supporting form of exercise, because it is probably the most pleasurable form of activity that burns calories. On the average, a good active sexual encounter burns about 200 calories. The emphasis is on "active" because you all know (we hope) that there is making love and there is *making love!* There is a saying in German: *"Ein guter Hahn wird selten fett,"* which means: A good rooster seldom gets fat. This is quite true, but when the rooster gets fat, his roostering will slow down tremendously.

WHERE TO EXERCISE

This is probably one of the most important decisions you can make.

When was the last time that you went out and bought some exercise equipment? How often did you use it before it wound up in a closet or in the garage? The point I am trying to make is that nobody really likes to exercise at home and/or alone.

One of the joys of exercising is that we can do it together with other people, or that we have a chance to meet people who have the same interests. A sport like volleyball is ideal; it gives us exercise and brings us together with others. Of course, this is not usually an all-year-round activity.

So where are you going to exercise? To some degree this will depend on the climate in your area. Extreme hot or cold climates often make strenuous outdoor exercise impossible. Many types of exercises have moved indoors. YMCAs, gyms, and a variety of health clubs have everything from swimming pools to exercise-equipment rooms and areas for jazz-nastics and other aerobic activities.

Can you discipline yourself enough to do your exercise routine all by yourself, or would it be better to join a club where you are guided by trained instructors or where exercise classes are run by competent teachers? Naturally, if you decide to join any kind of club, money for your membership plays a role. Think about it before you sign a contract. Compare, and make sure that what you pay for is really what you want.

If you consider becoming a member in a health club, you should evaluate all long and short-term possibilities. Is the club you consider joining a small local enterprise? Is it associated with other clubs, just in case you move or get transferred? Do their hours of operation suit you?

There are an infinite variety of ways to exercise. After all, there are an infinite variety of personalities and people. Find an exercise program that you enjoy as much as possible.

EXERCISE SHOWS

When you work hard at losing weight and your bathroom scale tells you that you haven't lost an ounce, don't give up. This will happen frequently to people who go on a strong exercise program but haven't exercised in a long time.

What really happens is that the weight loss in fat is balanced by a gain in lean muscle mass. Muscle mass weighs more than fat, and therefore, the negative results (according to your bathroom scale) should not really disturb you. Under these conditions a more precise indicator of your health/appearance would be a bathroom mirror.

If you had taken a photo of yourself before you started your new health regimen (suggested by many weight-loss professionals), you would now see that your body has been reshaped. The different improvements would be obvious. A great decrease in body fat would show.

AN EXPERIMENT IN "LIFE EXTENSION"

When *Life Extension*, the Durk Pearson and Sandy Shaw best-seller, appeared in the book stores, I took a look at it and, at first glance, it seemed good to me. It contained lots of material, nothing new for the expert but possibly very interesting to the layperson. However, since more and more people asked about the various ideas in this book, I decided to take a closer look.

The authors suggest that sniffing Diapid will stimulate the body to grow muscles. Diapid contains vasopressin, which is supposed to stimulate the pituitary to release growth hormones. The importance of exercise is therefore played down. This simplistic "logic" can bring an exercise-physiologist's blood to the boiling point. Having written a book about aging, I am now constantly bombarded with questions about the Pearson-Shaw ideas.

Since I am a very strong exercise enthusiast myself, I decided to perform two experiments. In the first experiment, there were no differences between the life spans of the animals treated with Diapid and the control group. The controls received only distilled water instead of the drug. After four months of treating adult animals with the drug, the control group showed a slightly longer average life span; we then terminated the study.

In the second experiment, I used myself as a guinea pig. Over a four-week period, I sniffed Diapid (at a cost of $100 per month); almost all my exercise, except for a small maintenance program, was deliberately stopped. My body fat was measured by Dr. Frank Katch's method, before and after this experiment. After the four weeks I gained nine pounds of fat and lost about four pounds of lean muscle mass, my body fat changed from 13.8 percent to 19.7 percent. I became very moody and decided to stop the experiment at this point.

I have only one suggestion for readers: Forget the gimmicks and stick to a proven aggressive regimen of good health practices and supernutrition. Just recently, in a JAMA article by Dr. Dean Ornish, the effectiveness of good health practices was reconfirmed.

The article backs up what we have said all along—sound health practices are very effective in preventing heart disease and other diseases.

WHAT HAPPENS IF YOU DON'T EXERCISE?

When you only reduce your intake of calories without exercising, your body starts to tear down lean muscle mass. Since calories are burned mainly in the muscles, even during times when you actually don't use them, this causes an overall decrease in your metabolism so that you now have to eat even less in order to prevent a weight gain. If you reduce your caloric intake even further, your body tears down more lean muscle mass and you go into a never-ending vicious cycle. You would have to eat less and less, weight loss would become more and more difficult, and since this will also affect your brain chemistry, your chances of becoming depressed would increase.

The only way to prevent this cycle is by exercising and building some muscle mass. As you have seen in the example given at the end of chapter 2, a weight-loss program that is combined with exercise will not only make you shed pounds, but will also build lean muscle mass at the same time.

CELLULITE, MORE THAN JUST A NEW NAME FOR AN OLD, FAMILIAR PROBLEM

A veterinarian once told me that even cows have cellulite. When farmers wanted to sell an older animal, they used to fatten it up to give it a healthy appearance. In some of these animals the underlying muscle that had given it the well-rounded shape disappeared, and when fattened up, the skin became rippled and cellulitelike. Veterinarians found that fibers that connected the skin to underlying muscle and bone were still there, but the excess fat had blown up the skin past its normal size. The connective fibers pulled the skin inward in some places. The farmers had veterinarians cut the connective fibers under the skin with fine surgical tools, which eliminated the rippled skin. (That's why my veterinarian friend always insisted that plastic surgery was actually discovered by cow doctors.)

The cellulite story in humans is very much the same. As we grow up, determined by genetics, the body builds a certain amount of muscle mass. Exercise just shapes these muscles a little bit, but it doesn't change the structure of the muscle groups. The nice, round, and "saftig" shape of a maybe even slightly overweight young woman is therefore due to a good amount of underlying muscle mass, covered with more or less fat, and held in the right place by stringlike fibers that connect skin, muscles, and bones.

If you have grown up in America, you probably haven't had any physical activities involving your whole body. Any one specific activity uses only a certain number of muscles, letting other muscle groups deteriorate. Whether you go to work, or to college, if you sit most of the time, more muscle mass is lost, and weight gain becomes a fact of life. After a few weight-loss attempts that usually don't include good exercises, you will have lost a lot of muscle mass, the stuff that gives you a nice shape, and fat has taken its place. Everything sags, and the remaining connective fibers pull the skin inward, giving it the rippled appearance that is now called cellulite. (See Fig. 7.3).

There must be a two-part approach to getting rid of cellulite: Lose the fat and rebuild the underlying muscle tissue. Most women are not successful because they either don't exercise or they just do one specific exercise, building only one of the many muscle groups. There are a large number of muscles in the thighs and the buttocks, and it takes a large number of exercises to rebuild all of them. If cellulite is your

Figure 7.3. Muscle Mass

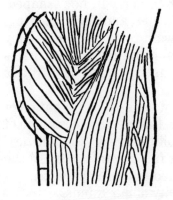

Well-toned muscle mass

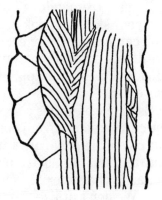

Loss of lean muscle
mass and gain of
fat (cellulite)

problem, be prepared for a long recovery program that includes many different exercises. Should you get the urge to quit, remember that nothing else works. In respect to nutrition, do everything that favors muscle formation.

A PROMISE

If you follow this program for just a few weeks, your spirits will greatly improve, and your stamina and overall energy will get a tremendous boost. Your figure will be reshaped, and your skin will look healthier, firmer, and not so sagging. You can choose the exercises you want to do, as long as they fulfill the requirements outlined. So choose any activity that is fun for you. Body shaping is a new part of the physical-fitness movement.

Each one of us has a specific set of genes, a combination of the chromosomes from our parents, that determines much of our physical appearance and possibilities. I say "possibilities" because most of us are not taking full advantage of all the fantastic characteristics we inherited from our parents.

1. We don't utilize the full capacity of our minds.

2. We let our bodies deteriorate; we put on weight and our bellies get bigger and bigger.

3. We get lazy and we drop out.

Whatever point you are at today, you can take charge of your own life and change all that. You will walk tall and proud again, in charge of your body. You can do it with exercise. You will lose weight, and you will shape up. But this is only the first step.

Body-Shaping
There are hundreds of muscles in your body that you never see and have probably never heard of, but it is these muscles, on top of your skeletal structure, that give your body its shape. If you use the correct exercise machines in a gym, these muscles can be increased or decreased in size to give you a more appealing overall appearance.

The easiest structural change for men and women to make

is to build up chest size and reduce hip circumference. (For more details, talk to an instructor at a good gym.)

If you don't believe that this can be done with *your* figure, check the "before" and "after" pictures of people in *Redesign Your Body: The 90-Day Real Body Makeover* by Drs. Anita and Franco Columbu.

REJUVENATING THE FACE WITH WRINKLE CHASERS

The "old" look that one's face gets is due to three major factors.

1) Overall aging. In agreement with several theories of aging, the causes of aging in the skin are not much different from the aging process on other parts of the body. Therefore, our anti-aging measures, detailed in chapter 16, also apply for slowing down the aging process of the skin. The greatest success in delaying further aging can probably be achieved with the use of anti-oxidants, which are already included in the recommended supplements. Limiting your exposure to sunlight, or at least using a good sunscreen lotion, is also important. Weight loss and overall improved health, the goal of our program, also leads to a younger and more radiant facial appearance.

2) A direct correlation between an "old" looking face and a lack of use of facial muscles is also established. Facial exercises (making faces) for about five to ten minutes per day can almost totally eliminate this self-induced aging factor.

3) There is also a direct correlation between moisture-retention and a "glowing," young-looking face. This is a science in itself. The cosmetics industry has developed a number of humectants (factors that attract moisture) for use in skin lotions. Most recently a connection between a compound in the skin (sodium salts of pyrrolidone carboxylic acid, NaPCA) and water retention was established. NaPCA is a truly fascinating substance that has a potential of being the ultimate wrinkle chaser. Researchers have established that NaPCA decreases in the skin as we age. Giving it back to the skin, via skin lotions, increases the skin's capacity to retain

moisture. Most cosmetics companies are scrambling to include this compound, together with other established humectants, to produce the ultimate skin product. As of the writing of this book, a check with major drugstore chains confirmed that only one company, VitaPlus Industries of Las Vegas, had a market-ready NaPCA skin lotion. The scientific references for research dealing with NaPCA have been included in the appendix.

A number of doctors have developed facial rejuvenation methods that can be combined with our weight-loss program. At our Health Integration Center, Dr. Christina Choi combines electrical stimulation of facial muscles with herbs, the NaPCA cream, and possibly acupuncture. Already after about five sessions one can see small wrinkles disappear and larger ones smooth out.

If, after you have followed a weight-loss and body-shaping program, you find that you still don't have the figure you'd like, there is still another step you can take. Recently, a new method, suction fat removal, has received much attention. It is a method that is usually done by a plastic surgeon, and it can be done on an outpatient basis.

A CASE HISTORY

A very determined 34-year-old woman who had participated in different sports all her life came to see me about weight loss and body shaping. She was also a runner and, despite all the exercise she was doing, her abdomen and legs showed a sizable amount of cellulite. Runners usually don't do sufficient upper-body (chest and arms) exercises. Over a six-week period, we were able to increase her upper-body size a little, and she was also able to lose nine pounds. Her proportions looked a little better in clothes, but in a swimsuit the picture was less encouraging.

After a visit with a Chicago cosmetic and youth surgeon, Dr. John Drammis, she decided to have the suction fat removal done. She was very happy with the results. The incisions necessary to do this are extremely small, and even in a swimsuit, one would have to point them out in order to notice them.

NOW GO TO FIGURE 10.1 AND CHECK ITEM 7

Decide how much exercising you are willing to do. You should now understand that weight loss without at least a minimum amount of physical activity is impossible. You have two choices.

1. You can do the absolute minimum of physical activity that will help maintain lean muscle tissue and that will burn *some* calories (walking, some aerobic exercises, fast dancing, etc., belong in this class). Please understand that these minor exercises are not enough to achieve the best possible health.

2. You can do exercises to achieve the best possible health, which will also reduce disease risks. Any exercise is all right if it is: done at least three times per week, done 30 minutes to 40 minutes each time without interruptions, and vigorous. "Vigorous" means that your pulse rate will reach the correct range, as discussed in this chapter.

For a person new to exercise, we have included a list of the DO's and DON'T's of exercise in appendix C.

8

WHEN STRESS BECOMES DISTRESS: How it affects eating habits and nutritional requirements and induces hunger mechanisms.

Reporter, interviewing a general: "With all the pressure and responsibilities in your job, don't you get any ulcers?"
The general: "I don't get ulcers. I give ulcers."

CHECK YOURSELF

When stress changes to distress, it becomes a major disease risk factor. We are all familiar with the picture of a man who, while under distress, clasps his chest and has a heart attack. According to the stress theory on aging, and well supported by medical research, distress is a definite life-shortening factor. In people with eating disorders, stress management becomes a number one priority. Most important, distress can seriously affect our eating by inducing a hunger mechanism.

1. Do you feel that, in your own definition, stress often "gets to you?" YES NO
2. When under stress, do you frequently visit your refrigerator? YES NO

3. Do you have an eating disorder
   such as bulimia?   YES   NO

If you answered "NO" to all three questions, you can check "Doesn't apply" for item 8 in Figure 10.1 and move on to the next chapter.

Going on a weight-loss program and learning how to take charge of your own life does subject you to a number of stress factors. This could be the most determining factor in reaching your weight-loss goal. Obviously, if you can't handle the distress that is associated with the changes you are required to make to lose weight, you will quit the program. We must prevent this!

Distress is your enemy, and the best way to fight an enemy is to get to know it; know where it comes from, how strong it is, and what it can do to you.

Professor Hans Selye said, "Reach always for your highest attainable aim, but never put up resistance in vain." This is exactly what this book is all about. I want you to be able to reach your goal with the least amount of distress. It can be done.

THE STRESS THEORY ON AGING

There is stress around us everywhere. If we can handle it, we can thrive on it and even get an extra boost from it. We achieve something important despite many obstacles (the stressors) and then savor the feeling of victory, enjoying the boost that comes from knowing that we were able to reach our goal.

If we can't handle it, if we are helpless or don't know what to do, if we just grind our teeth and talk to ourselves instead of to others, then stress changes and becomes distress, a negative force in our lives. According to Professor Selye, stress is a major cause of aging. When stress becomes distress, then we have moved to the losing side.

In numerous experiments on animals and humans, Professor Selye has repeatedly demonstrated the harmful effects of distress on health and aging. However, he also has demonstrated that winning a victory over distress is nothing but taking a number of logical steps and that the first step is to get to know the distress. Then, we can take countermeasures; and soon, we will be able to handle it automatically.

One experiment that Professor Selye performed involved a rat in a metal cage. Every time a light was turned on, the animal received a small shock, resulting in distress. This experiment was repeated with a wooden platform placed in the cage. The rat soon learned that by jumping on the wooden block when the light went on, it could avoid the shock. There were no long-term negative effects on this animal at all. In addition, there were many indications that such learned experiences actually improved the animal's health and made it live longer.

By using humans in the following example, we hope to show you how to overcome stress. For instance, assume that you take a back road to get to work. One day, a large hole appears and you drive your car right through this hole. Your car rattles and shakes, and you too are also quite shook up. A stressful situation.

The next day as you approach the road you may be concerned that the same thing will happen, but because you take the correct evasive action, you avoid hitting the hole. Avoiding the hole now becomes a routine move, and it becomes an unimportant factor in your life.

Some people might even make a game out of it and get a kick out of being able to avoid the hole. They are letting the stressor in their life know that they can handle it.

Now let's take a look at the holes in your road toward a desired weight.

IDENTIFYING THE STRESSORS

The largest stressor in people who want to lose weight is the worry that their efforts might not be successful and that all of these efforts are just too much to handle. Do you see the defeatist's attitude in that?

By determining precisely the important factors in *your* weight-loss program, we reduce the overall effort to an absolute minimum. In this program, you are also not taking any risks, such as taking dangerous diet drugs that might not work; everything you do will improve your health, your looks, and your longevity. So, you have nothing to worry about.

Physical activity, especially for people who are not used to exercising, might be considered a stressor. However, in reality, this is not so. It's been demonstrated that physical activity actually reduces hunger feelings and strengthens the body so that it is in a much better position to deal with distress. Again, you are in charge and well prepared.

How will you be able to handle your bad moods, depression, and "down" feelings, together with the stress of all.the things you are supposed to do in this weight-loss program? Stop this negative thinking! The exercise alone will improve your mood and help rid you of any depression. You should discipline yourself to follow the program for about four weeks. The results will be so dramatic that it will boost your confidence tremendously!

All we have to do is convince *you* that *you* can do it. It can be done. You can do it. The actual doing is easy!

STRESS RAISES YOUR NUTRITIONAL REQUIREMENTS

When you are put under stress, your body goes into overdrive to deal with the stress situation. Your blood pressure increases, your adrenalin starts flowing, and blood-clotting reactions are initiated. All this involves the use of the nutrients that you absorbed from your diet.

These mechanisms for handling stress are pretty well researched and established. Hundreds of research projects have evaluated the body's nutritional requirements when under stress, and the findings show that we need more B vitamins and vitamin C. That's why you see all those commercials about stress vitamins on television.

But the quality of foods must also be good. Any change toward lower-than-acceptable standards reduces the body's capacity to deal with stress; sugar in the diet is especially detrimental.

Dealing with the nutritional requirements for combatting stress is easy. We have already discussed the quality of foods and food composition, and the B vitamins and vitamin C are already included in the supplementation program. Distress also activates carbohydrate hunger mechanisms and induces cravings for sweets.

SUFFICIENT SLEEP—ANOTHER DISTRESS EQUALIZER

Studies in gerontology (aging research) have focused on the amount of sleep required for the best possible health and longevity. Such studies have shown that the longest life span is achieved with an average of seven hours to eight hours of sleep per night. Naturally, our most basic goal is to enjoy life. We can do it better if we are alert, well rested, and full of energy. Deviations, too much or too little sleep, induce distress in our body in different ways.

Earlier we mentioned how important it is to exercise at least three times per week. This takes time, and if you have a regular job, your time is probably limited. Add to this other things that you have to do, from laundry to handling personal affairs, and time becomes a key factor. This is a reality you must face.

An exercise program, done after work, takes a lot out of you and the need for rest will be increased. A common sense approach would be to try to exercise on days when you have made no other plans. Afterward, relax, watch TV, and go to bed at a reasonable hour. You'll wake up feeling refreshed. The next day can be devoted to enjoying life and good company. When you are rested and alert, you can handle anything. Worries are reduced to a minimum.

LEARN TO MEDITATE

When you come home from work, when you relax from a hectic day, before you go out on a date, or whenever you have thirty minutes for yourself, you can do something magnificent for yourself—meditate.

There are many ways to meditate, and it's easy to learn. You can do it standing up, sitting, or lying down. Here is just one way that I find relaxing, and it also gives me a tremendous recharge.

Turn off everything, from radio to TV and telephone. Then lie on your back on a comfortable couch or bed. Close your eyes, relax, and think of some nice, positive things. Now comes the main part of the relaxing–meditating. Starting with your feet, you search for tense spots in your body, and you imagine that you drain the tension through the bottom of your heels.

Now you move up to your calves, search for tense spots, and drain the tension through the bottom of your heels.

You do the same thing for your entire body, moving upward to your knees, your thighs, abdomen, chest, arms, neck, and head.

Do it step by step: relax, search for the tense spots, and each time drain the tension through the bottom of your feet.

Often I don't even make it up to my chest before I am asleep. A short nap like this, lasting for fifteen to thirty minutes at a time, is refreshing and gives you a recharge.

Try it! I bet you'll like it.

NOW GO TO FIGURE 10.1 AND CHECK ITEMS 7 AND 8

If you have determined that stress is a major factor in your life, there are basically three things you can do: exercise, take stress vitamins, and plan your daily activities well so that you get enough rest.

1. If you already have a strong exercise program, there is no need to increase exercise even further. If you are only doing a minimum amount of physical activity (7a), then we hope that you will move up to the next exercise level (7b).

2. B vitamins and vitamin C are already included in our recommendations for supplementation. Only if you had earlier, after chapter 4, decided not to take supplements, should you reconsider now.

3. Planning your daily activities to reduce stress and to make certain that you are doing all you can is a key point in the stress-reducing program. You might even go a step further and consider taking a stress-management seminar or read a book about stress; we recommend *Stress Without Distress* by Professor Hans Selye.

9

LOW BLOOD-SUGAR PROBLEMS: How they can make your body scream for food and make your weight-loss program a failure.

> Like opium, morphine, and heroin, sugar is an addictive, destructive drug, yet Americans consume it daily in everything from cigarettes to bread. If you are overweight, or suffer from migraine, hypoglycemia, or acne, the plague of the Sugar Blues has hit you. In fact, by accepted diagnostic standards, our entire society is prediabetic.
>
> William Duffy
> Author of *Sugar Blues*

CHECK YOURSELF

Here, we'll check to see if you have a possible blood-sugar problem and/or a special insulin sensitivity, and we'll explain how consumption of sweets can induce depression and premature aging. It can also induce extreme hunger and a craving for more sweets and totally prevent your body from burning fat.

1. Do you often have a craving for sweets, even sweet fruits?   YES   NO
2. Is it difficult for you to lose weight even if you exercise and reduce your overall food intake?   YES   NO

125

3. Is your score more than 35 points
   on the Harper Health Indicator
   Test? (See Fig. 9.1.)   YES   NO

If you answered "NO" to all three questions, you can check "Doesn't apply" for item 9 in Table 10.1 and start reading chapter 10.

Low blood-sugar problems have been established as major heart disease and diabetes risks, and they can also make a weight-loss program nightmarish, keeping you hungry all the time while preventing your body from burning off fat successfully. It can lead to nervousness, shaking, blackouts, depression, self-deprecating thoughts, and more serious mental disorders if not stopped in time. In the treatment of binging and mental disorders, dealing with low blood-sugar levels is the first and most important step in a successful recovery program.

Many professionals in the holistic and preventive medical field believe that these are not "real" medical disorders; instead, it is the excessive consumption of the wrong foods, combined with other faulty health practices, that induces low blood-sugar levels. The validity of this kind of thinking, namely, that faulty nutrition and the wrong health practices can bring on diseases and that the right nutrition and health practices can cure diseases, has been supported by the medical literature.

DO YOU SUFFER FROM HYPOGLYCEMIA?

Dr. Harold Harper past president of the International Academy of Preventive Medicine and president of the American Academy of Medical Preventics, practicing in North Hollywood, California, designed a simple test (Fig. 9.1) that can be used as an indicator of health.

Listed below are the ratings for your chances of having a blood-sugar disorder. If yours exceeds 75 percent, incorporating the right nutritional action is a harmless way toward greatly improving your weight-loss approach.

Ratings:

20 points or less:	Your chance is only about 5 percent or less of having an abnormal glucose-tolerance level.
20–25 points:	Probability increases to 50 percent.
25–35 ponts:	Probability increases to 75 percent.
35–45 points:	Your probability of having an abnormal glucose-tolerance level increases to 90 percent.
45 points or more:	Probability is 98 percent or more.

HYPOGLYCEMIA (LOW BLOOD-SUGAR LEVEL)

This is a very serious disorder that, if not corrected, can ultimately lead to depression, anxiety, and diabetes.

Your body's major fuel is glucose (blood sugar), and it has several mechanisms that serve to maintain blood-sugar homeostasis (normal blood-sugar levels within reasonable limits). Blood-sugar deviations from these normal ranges, too high or too low, will throw your body into physiological imbalances. High blood-sugar levels, hyperglycemia or diabetes, is usually preceded by hypoglycemia, along with a battery of warning signals ranging from fainting spells to cravings for sweets, weight gain, and depression.

Do you have any idea how bad excess sugar can be for you? If you have difficulty giving up sweets, unbrainwash yourself and read *Sugar Blues* by William Duffy. It will change your mind!

How do we get hypoglycemia? The mechanism is very simple. When maintaining "normal" blood-sugar levels, our body utilizes the capacity of the liver and lean muscle mass to store slight excesses of ingested carbohydrates in the form of glycogen. Carbohydrates are digested and become glucose; glucose stored in the liver and lean muscle mass is called glycogen. When we talk about slight excesses of carbohydrates, we mean those amounts that are not being burned immediately to give energy. Energy calories come from all foods, and therefore, the total amount of calories consumed is important.

Figure 9.1. Harper Health Indicator Test

Take this test now. Do not check your score until later. Check off each symptom that you have according to its severity.

- (0) means you never have the symptom,
- (1) means it is mild when it occurs or it occurs occasionally,
- (2) means moderate or occurring at least once a week, and
- (3) means severe or occurring frequently.

0	1	2	3	
				Tired all the time
				Hungry between meals or at night
				Depressed
				Insomnia
				Wake up after a few hours sleep
				Fearful (overwhelmed by people, places, or things)
				Can't decide easily
				Can't concentrate
				Poor memory
				Worry frequently
				Feel insecure or low self-image
				Highly emotional
				Moody
				Cry easily, or feel like crying inside
				Fits of anger
				Magnify insignificant details (make mountains out of molehills)
				Eat candy, cake, cookies, or drink soda pop
				Eat bread, pasta, potatoes, rice, or beans
				Consume alcohol
				Drink more than 3 cups of coffee or cola drinks daily
				Crave candy, soda, or coffee between meals or mid-afternoon
				Can't work well under pressure
				Headaches
				Sleepy during the day
				Sleepy or drowsy after meals

	Lack of energy
	Reduced initiative
	Can't get started in the morning
	Eat when nervous
	Stomach cramps or "nervous stomach"
	Allergies: asthma, hay fever, skin rash, sinus trouble, etc.
	Fatigue relieved by eating
	Suicidal thoughts or tendencies, feelings of hopelessness
	Bored
	Bad dreams
	Irritable before meals
	Heart beats fast (palpitations)
	Get shaky inside if hungry
	Feel faint if meal is delayed
	Ulcers, gastritis, chronic indigestion, abdominal bloating
	Cold hands or feet
	Trembling (shaking) of the hands
	Blurred vision
	Bleeding gums
	Dizziness, giddiness, or light-headedness
	Aware of breathing heavily
	Bruise easily
	Reduced sex drive
	Incoordination (drop or bump into things)
	Sweating excessively
	Unsocial or anti-social behavior
	Muscle twitching or cramps
	Excessive thirst
	Phobias
	Weight change
	Frequent urination
	TOTAL*

*Multiply the number of checks in each column by the number at the top of the column and then add the numbers in the three columns to get your total score.

Note: From *How You Can Beat the Killer Diseases,* by Harold Harper

Also, if you are not very physically active, there is no need for your body to burn lots of calories.

We consume two types of carbohydrates, refined and complex. Complex carbohydrates, such as vegetables, whole-grain products, and fruits, are digested *slowly* and produce glucose. Refined carbohydrates, usually from white-flour products and sweets, are digested fast and produce glucose, and the blood-sugar level changes rapidly.

Usually a sedentary life-style, in combination with an excessive intake of calories in general, and sugars and sweets specifically, causes rapidly changing blood-sugar levels. The body reacts to bring the blood-sugar level back to normal; insulin is released by the pancreas. Since the physical-activity level is low, liver and lean muscle mass storage capacity for glucose is limited or not available at all. So an excess of sugar is converted to fat. Under such extreme conditions, the pancreas often overreacts and the blood-sugar level falls below normal. This induces a craving for sweets and more food, and the cycle starts again. If this cycle is not interrupted, blood-sugar imbalances get worse, the cravings for sweets increase, weight increases, and mood changes occur. Also, the low blood-sugar levels change the brain chemistry and depression is induced; irritability, shaking, dizziness, fainting spells, and blackouts become more serious. When this insulin mechanism finally breaks down, the opposite condition, hyperglycemia or diabetes, occurs.

Reducing overall food intake, especially fats and sugar, and consuming more complex carbohydrates such as vegetables and whole-grain products, greatly slows down the rate at which glucose is fed into the bloodstream; blood-sugar level changes become less dramatic.

Increasing one's physical activity not only burns up more calories, but it also creates more lean muscle mass, which increases the body's capacity to store glucose. Lean muscle mass actually serves as a buffer against blood-sugar imbalances.

How can we interrupt the cycle? Adjustments in one or both of the above areas can give immediate results.

All signs associated with hypoglycemia disappear rapidly.

A NUMBER OF THEORIES ON AGING SUPPORT THE IMPORTANCE OF MAINTAINING NORMAL BLOOD-SUGAR LEVELS

The theories range from the cybernetic theory to my "Combination Theory on Aging" to various aspects of aging research that is presently going on under the direction of some of the leading researchers at MIT.

A little science for the person who wants to know "why?"
When the blood-sugar level is low, the body converts amino acids to glucose to keep the blood-sugar level within reasonable ranges. This then causes an imbalance between amino acids in the blood; tryptophan remains at whatever level it was, but phenylalanine and tyrosine are much lower. Mood and aging-associated chemicals in the brain are made from these amino acids; tryptophan is converted to serotonin, and phenylalanine and tyrosine are changed to norepinephrine and dopamine. The imbalance of the amino acids in the blood now leads to an imbalance of these neurotransmitters in the brain. The medical literature has associated these imbalances with depression and premature aging.

The prevention of blood-sugar disorders, from temporary, self-induced hypoglycemia to advanced hypoglycemia, is therefore of the greatest importance in the prevention of chronic diseases and aging.

Refined-carbohydrate intake: (sugar, sweets, white-flour products)	Blood-sugar level goes up rapidly. Pancreas responds and releases too much insulin. Blood-sugar level is brought down to below normal.
	RESULTS: Cravings for sweets. Amino acids, possibly from lean muscle mass, are changed to glucose. Glucose is changed to fat.

Complex-Carbohydrate intake: Blood-sugar level rises slowly.
(vegetables, whole-grain   Part of the glucose is burned as
products, fruits)   fuel, and the body has enough
                                 time to store any excess glucose
                                 in the liver and lean muscle
                                 mass. No need for the pancreas
                                 to release excess insulin or for
                                 glucose to be converted to fat.

A CASE HISTORY

After I spoke at one of the preventive medicine meetings, a doctor came up to me and asked if I could possibly talk to one of his patients, a woman who, despite rigid exercise and a good nutritional program, was unsuccessful in losing twenty extra pounds.

When I met with her later, I was going to suggest all kinds of measures, from an evaluation of all her health practices and nutrition to blood analysis, and so forth, but discovered this had already been done; her doctor was very thorough. She told me that several months ago, she had gone to see her doctor to discuss a weight-loss program. She was already practicing good nutrition and had a good exercise program; therefore, only minor adjustments had to be made. She did not, however, lose the weight.

A computerized nutrition evaluation showed that she was on a 1,700-calorie diet. For her level of activity and ideal weight, this was already very low.

More nutritional adjustments were made. Her caloric intake was lowered to 1,400 calories per day. The woman stayed on the program for several weeks but lost only about two pounds. Also, she was feeling weak and irritable. This didn't make any sense.

The woman was about 5 feet 7 inches tall, and a stress test showed that she was in good physical shape. Feeling weak and irritable, with blood analysis showing triglycerides in a normal range, suggested that extreme measures should not be taken. But I certainly didn't want to tell her to keep the extra twenty pounds and try to be happy.

I decided to take a closer look at her diet. It looked pretty good. There were some very small amounts of refined carbohydrates in the form of carrot cake and other desserts, but the amount of calories was so small that it shouldn't have had any bad effect. Upon still closer examination of a so-called natural cereal, I found that it really wasn't natural and had too much sugar in it. We also found several other foods that had hidden sugar in them.

We decided to eliminate *all* the sugar and refined carbohydrates from the diet, including the carrot cake and desserts. It worked! The extra pounds came off rapidly, and she was even able to go to a higher overall caloric intake while still losing weight. Why did it work?

THE SUGAR-INSULIN-FAT CONNECTION

It has long been known that insulin stimulates the conversion of glucose to fat in the adipose tissue. The presence of insulin also keeps the fat in the fat cells and prevents utilization of fats. In other words, despite the presence of small amounts of insulin, most people metabolize carbohydrates, fats, and protein at the same time. However, some people apparently have an extreme insulin sensitivity that almost totally blocks the utilization of fat. This means that even a small amount of sugar will cause the pancreas to release enough insulin to totally block the metabolism and burning of fat.

Does your weight-loss condition sound similar to the one described in our case history? Have you tried to lose weight by cutting down on the overall number of calories you consume, without removing all refined carbohydrates, and been totally unsuccessful in losing weight? You may have this insulin sensitivity.

If this is the case, you should not only remove all refined carbohydrates from your diet, but you should also put sweet fruits on your hit list. For some people this would be like asking them to give up the love of their lives.

Talking about life, do you want to live? How do you want to live? Why not give it a try for a few weeks? It certainly won't hurt you.

Then, you can still decide what is more important in your life: some sugar consumption or your health and gorgeous figure.

TRY TO UNDERSTAND YOUR BODY

Most people understand why their automobiles need tune-ups, lubrication, and oil, and they seem to take care of their automobiles better than their bodies. Maybe this is because they don't understand the functioning of their bodies.

When we consume carbohydrates, they wind up in the bloodstream as glucose. If the blood-glucose level rises, the glucose is stored in the liver and in the lean muscle mass as glycogen. Much of this occurs in response to insulin released by the pancreas. Insulin controls blood-sugar levels, and it opens the doors of the cells so that glucose can get in. If the blood-sugar level rises even further—as in the case when you have excess sugar in the diet—the pancreas releases even more insulin and the excess sugar in the blood now gets into the adipose tissue and is converted into fat. This chemical process in the body is relatively fast and easy, but the opposite—removal of fat from the fat tissue—is more complicated (Fig. 9.2).

In order to get rid of the extra fat on your body, first, the caloric intake must be restricted so that the body is forced to use some of the stored energy (fat). Then, the fat is taken apart into it's basic building blocks: the fatty acids and glycerol. The next step is to release the fatty acids back into the bloodstream so that they can be transported to the cells that do the burning of fat. However, as you can see in Figure 9.3, insulin blocks the utilization of the stored fat. Any sugar in the diet that stimulates the pancreas to release excess insulin prevents the body from burning fat. In some people this insulin sensi-

Figure 9.2. Normal Pathways of Foods in Your Body—with extra sugar in the diet.

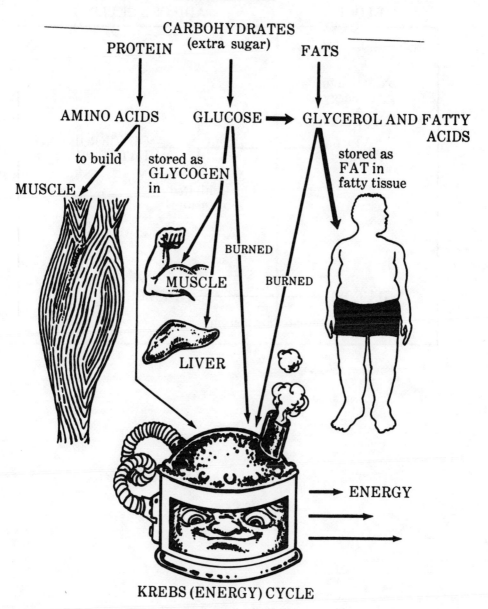

FOOD INTAKE

CARBOHYDRATES
(extra sugar)

PROTEIN   FATS

AMINO ACIDS   GLUCOSE ➤ GLYCEROL AND FATTY ACIDS

to build   stored as GLYCOGEN in   stored as FAT in fatty tissue

MUSCLE

BURNED

MUSCLE

BURNED

LIVER

ENERGY

KREBS (ENERGY) CYCLE

Figure 9.3. How Insulin, Released Through Sugar Intake, Prevents the Body from Burning Fat.

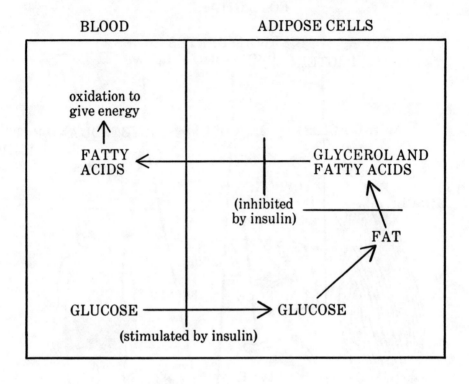

tivity is so severe that even the strictest caloric restrictions are ineffective as long as there is some sugar in the diet that stimulates the pancreas to release excess insulin.

There is no precise way of predicting if you have such an insulin sensitivity. However, eliminating all sugar, and even sweet fruit, from your diet, and replacing it with vegetables, greens, and other complex carbohydrates, will certainly do you no harm.

Data supporting the above findings and reasoning for weight loss were presented at the 1979 and 1981 meetings of the American College of Sports Medicine.

NOW GO TO FIGURE 10.1 AND CHECK ITEM 9

If you have a possible blood-sugar problem, there are four actions you can take. Some have been previously recommended. If they apply to you, make sure to place a star next to the action to indicate a high priority.

a) Exercise is important because it builds lean muscle mass, which serves as a buffer against blood-sugar imbalances. Remember, glucose is stored in the liver and lean muscle mass as glycogen. If you already have a good exercise program that fulfills the requirements for the best possible disease prevention, then, this point is unimportant for you.

b) Remove sugar and refined carbohydrates from your diet as much as you can. This is a very important action. If you have a special insulin sensitivity, removing *all* sugar (even sugar hidden in many foods) and sweet fruit is a must if you want your weight loss to be successful.

c) For people with blood-sugar disorders, having lean protein in every meal is of the greatest importance. You will also find it extremely helpful to include frequent, small amounts of a protein drink in your diet; for example, between breakfast and lunch, and in the afternoon.

d) take a GTF supplement. GTF is an organic chromium compound that helps normalize blood-sugar mechanisms. You can get it in health-food stores.

10

YOUR PERSONAL ANTI-AGING WEIGHT-LOSS PROFILE EMERGES. It pinpoints what you have to do to guarantee your easy weight loss.

> Combining several weight-loss factors can
> save you up to 1,500 calories per day, or the
> equivalent of three pounds per week.
> > University of Alabama School
> > of Medicine study, 1983

A CASE HISTORY

A few years ago, when I was living in Chicago, a man consulted me about his weight problem. In summary, here is what his daily routine was like. Until the previous year, his job kept him reasonably active and he would burn up the calories he consumed; his caloric intake was equal to his output even though he had no special exercise program.

Then, two things changed his life: He was promoted to a desk job, and he began dating a girl who had to work late. In the evening he would routinely wait for her to finish work, and then they would have a late-night dinner. His friend had a sweet tooth and often ordered some dessert; he liked it and joined in. So he started to gain weight. At first, he tried to cut down on foods a little, but it wasn't very effective. Then, he tried to sneak in some quick exercise before meeting his girlfriend, but that only made him tired and he often fell asleep early in the evening. Taking diet pills helped him somewhat, but when he stopped taking them (because they affected his mood), he gained weight even faster. He started to panic and that is when he decided to consult with me.

A major factor in his weight problem was his slowing metabolism (this is common with many people who reach the age of 30 or 35). When he was younger, his work-related physical activity enabled him to maintain a certain amount of lean muscle mass and burn up more calories. But because of his new job, he wasn't using his muscles, so they started to deteriorate. The late meals caused more problems, and the desserts sealed his fate. The excess calories, faulty eating habits, sugar, lack of physical activity, and the general slow-down of the metabolism was too much to be corrected by a small amount of exercise and some caloric reductions.

At first we used a computer method to check his overall nutrition. It showed that his fat content was very high. Slight adjustments in the choice of foods solved this problem. He agreed to cut out about half of the desserts. It just so happened that a neighborhood soccer team practiced on the two nights he didn't spend with his girlfriend. He liked soccer and joined the team; he got a really good workout on those two nights and had time to rest. On two other days, during his lunchtime, he went for a long walk. Then, when he got home, he had time to rest before he met his girlfriend, and they ate earlier.

All in all, we made four changes: adjustment of the general food intake (less fat), reduction of refined-carbohydrate calories (elimination of some desserts), increase in two types of physical activity (soccer and walking), and eating dinner earlier. This, in combination with the right amount of rest, did the trick. He lost the weight and became more health conscious.

Why do I relate this case history? Because it demonstrates our basic approach! By combining several weight-loss modalities, shedding pounds becomes easy. Also, an awareness of the many health- and weight-related factors helps you keep the weight off.

YOUR ANTI-AGING WEIGHT-LOSS PROFILE

At this point, having checked all the items in Figure 10.1, your personal anti-aging weight-loss profile should be complete. If there are any check marks in the column "Not sure," review some of the previous material and possibly use any one of the analytical methods recommended at the end of this chapter to clarify these points.

Take a look at Figure 10.1. The column "Important to do" points out what you have to do to shed pounds. Many items that apply to you give you a choice of actions you can take. If in doubt, plan to do a little bit more. In part 3 of this book, we'll teach you *how* to do it right without overlooking anything. But in order to get there, we must make sure that none of the possible weight-loss obstacles (part 2) stand in the path of your shedding those pounds. From here on, your weight-loss program becomes easier and easier.

Priorities—which actions to emphasize

Items 1 and 2 in Figure 10.1 are there to tune you in and demonstrate to you that your approach works. Item 6 is there as health and anti-aging insurance so that your body will be strong enough to do whatever is necessary. The remaining items give you the important basic weight-loss actions that will make the program a success. You have probably recognized that a certain action, such as exercising, reducing fat, or increasing lean protein, can be recommended more than once. If, in *your* personal anti-aging weight-loss profile, a certain action is suggested more than once, then, it is an important action for you to take, and it should have priority in your program.

For example, if exercise comes up three times in your personal anti-aging weight-loss profile, this should tell you that your weight-loss program will be very successful if you

Figure 10.1. Your Anti-Aging Weight-Loss Profile.

	Already doing	Important to do	Not sure	Doesn't apply
1. If low metabolism is indicated: a. Activate lean muscle mass with exercise.				
b. Possibly have thyroid checked by your doctor.				
2. a. Weigh yourself every morning.				
b. Record body measurements and possibly determine body fat every 7 days.				
3. Keep a simple nutrition log and: a. Make sure that your daily caloric intake is in the desired range.				
b. Compare your nutrition to our food charts (Tables 3.1–3.3) and record if any of the following changes are required: Reduce sugar (Table 3.3)				
Reduce fats (Table 3.3)				
Increase fiber (Table 3.1)				

Eat lean protein in every meal (Table 3.2)	
4. a. Further increase fiber (Table 3.1).	
b. Further reduce fats.	
5. a. Eat a good breakfast.	
b. Eat a small, quality lunch.	
c. Eat dinner not later than 6 P.M. or 7 P.M.	
6. Take vitamin and mineral supplements.	
7. Choose a physical activity program—check item a, item b, or item c. a. Minimum program.	
b. Strong, aggressive program.	
c. Do body-shaping exercises.	
8. Distress appears to be a major factor in your life; to counteract it: a. Exercise.	
b. Take B complex and vitamin C.	
c. Plan your days well and make sure to get enough rest.	
9. Possible blood-sugar problems and/or special insulin sensitivity. a. Exercise.	
b. Reduce sugar.	
c. Eat lean protein in every meal.	
d. Take GTF supplement.	

exercise and that it has little chance of being successful if you don't exercise.

To make certain that you have a clear understanding of what you have to do to lose weight, review the column "Important to do" in Figure 10.1 and write the recommended action in the space on the left in Figure 10.2.

Now, in the space on the right, list with colored pen any recommended action that has been noted more than once. Give these actions a certain priority in your program and never skip them. Most people would have no problem losing weight if they followed their priority actions exclusively, but to make losing weight more effective, it is better if you include some additional actions.

PROOF THAT COMBINING FACTORS GIVES MUCH BETTER RESULTS

A Nutrition Study

Researchers at the University of Alabama School of Medicine placed two groups of people—one lean, the other overweight—on two different diets and allowed them to eat until they felt satisfied. Both diets were prepared by experienced cooks so that people found them equally varied, attractive and palatable.

The "Clean" diet: People were allowed to choose from the following: fresh fruit, cereal with no sugar in it, skim milk, coffee or tea, soups, salads, fish, chicken, vegetables, whole-wheat rolls, and other low-fat foods.

The "Dirty" diet: People were allowed to choose from: fried eggs, bacon, fast foods, fried lunches, steak, whole milk, buttered vegetables, buttered toast, pie, ice cream, and so forth.

Results: Whether the people were overweight or lean, while they were on the "clean" diet, they consumed an average of 1,500 calories per day; however, while on the "dirty" diet, they consumed an average of 3,000 calories per day. The researchers also noted that the average 1,500 calories on the "clean" diet were about 300 calories per day above the daily caloric need (DCML) for people who don't exercise.

This research cleverly combined several factors that lead to

Figure 10.2 Recommended Actions

Recommended Action	*Action Recommended More than Once*
1) a)	
b)	
2) a)	
b)	
3) a)	
b)	
4) a)	
b)	
5) a)	
b)	
c)	
6)	
7) a)	
b)	
c)	
8) a)	
b)	
c)	
9) a)	
b)	
c)	
d)	

tremendous caloric savings, and that have been discussed in detail in this book. It also suggests that weight loss without a reasonable amount of physical activity is an impossibility.

In addition, eating the "clean" diet took 30 percent more eating time than eating the "dirty" diet took; that's one-third more time to eat half the calories. Taking longer to eat is good because it takes time for the stomach to send the "I am full" or "satiated" message to the brain. If you eat fast foods, you consume lots of calories in a short time, and by the time your stomach sends the "full" signal to the brain, you have over-stuffed yourself.

A Longevity Study

To show the combined effects of good and bad health factors on longevity, we studied two groups of animals. One group was subjected to the wrong things, such as extra sugar in the diet, unlimited food supply, no exercise, and cigarette smoke. The second group had the right things, such as exercise, limited food supply, no sugar in the diet, no cigarette smoke, and a number of vitamin and mineral supplements.

The results showed that the difference in the average life span between the two groups was close to 100 percent. The animals in the second group lived longer, were leaner, and also showed the external signs of aging much later in their lives.

The more anti-aging factors we combine, the longer the life span of any species. The same principle is true for weight loss; the more weight-loss factors you combine, the easier and faster your weight loss will be.

Successful weight-loss

Combining several modalities to give the best possible weight loss has been suggested by a number of researchers. Proof that such an approach works best and gives long-lasting results, was reported by Drs. R. Colvin, S. Olson, and L. Sheldahl.

Removal of toxic chemicals from the body

More than 90 percent of adults carry five or more toxic

chemicals in their bodies. These chemicals can affect everything from increasing your risk of cancer to affecting your sexual functioning and nervous system. A 30 percent decrease in male sperm count has been blamed on these toxic chemicals; there are predictions that the situation will get worse and that 40 percent of all men will be sterile by the year 2,000.

Organochlorine Residues in Human Adipose Tissue

Residue	*Frequency of detection, %*
Total DDT	100
trans-Nonachlor	97
Heptachlor epoxide	96
Oxychlordane	95
Dieldrin	95

A program very similar to our weight-loss approach, combining exercise, sweating (induced by exercise and the use of a sauna), supplementation (general and larger amounts of niacin), has been shown to remove up to 66 percent of these toxic chemicals from the body within two to three weeks. So, while you shed pounds on our anti-aging weight-loss program, you will also be ridding your body of some of those toxic chemicals.

Follow-up Procedures

Some people find it difficult to calculate their own caloric intake, estimate fat and protein intake, and so forth. All this can be done with simple computer techniques. A number of these computer programs even evaluate all of your health practices and calculate your risk age. See Appendix D.

Since minerals play such an important part in maintaining the best possible health, you might want to have them checked with a hair analysis. The mineral content of your hair is an excellent indication of how much mineral is absorbed by your body, which toxic minerals might affect your health, and whether or not you should take mineral supplements. Hair analysis, done by a reputable laboratory, is an extremely important new analytical method that should be used by every health professional. Since this book is not the place for a detailed discussion, we would like to recommend *Trace Elements, Hair Analysis and Nutrition* by Richard Passwater, Ph.D., and Elmer Cranton, M.D., for reading by the professional and educated layperson.

As demonstrated in chapter 13, extreme dietary habits can greatly affect the mineral content in your body; serious mineral deficiencies can be life-threatening.

To stay up-to-date about what is happening in the health field and weight-loss and aging research, we recommend that you subscribe to the Holistic and Preventive UP-DATE, the official newsletter of the International Academy of Holistic Health and Medicine.

If you can't get the hair analysis or the newsletter from your doctor or nutritionist, check Appendix D for more details.

Part 2

Obstacles that Could Make Your Weight-Loss Program a Failure

Life itself is the proper binge.

Julia Child

11

HIGH-CALORIE DRINKS: Not just alcoholic drinks.

> About 112,000 women in the United States are expected to be diagnosed as having breast cancer. According to a study of hospitalized women in the United States, Canada, and Israel, women who drink [alcoholic beverages] regularly—at least four days a week—have 2 to 3½ times the risk of nondrinkers of getting breast cancer.
>
> *Lancet*, January 1983

CHECK YOURSELF

Excess liquid calories, consumed in the form of nonalcoholic and/or alcoholic beverages, can be a major obstacle in a person's weight-loss program. People sometimes believe that liquids can't be converted to something more substantial such as fat. In some cases people drink more than fifty percent of their daily caloric requirement, and when asked about their daily caloric intake, they only count food calories. Under such conditions the overall intake of important nutrients is greatly reduced, and nutrition becomes substandard.

1. Do you consume high-calorie beverages such as regular soda, coffee or tea sweetened with sugar, or

other sweetened drinks on a regu-
lar basis (2 or more per day)?   YES   NO

2. Do you drink more than one alco-
holic beverage per day?   YES   NO

3. Do all your combined daily liquid
calories account for more than 300
calories for a small person—120 lbs
or less), or 500 calories (for a larger
person)?   YES   NO

If you answered "NO" to at least items 1 and 3 or 2 and 3, you
can skip this chapter; otherwise, you should read this chapter.

HOW MUCH WEIGHT DO YOU DRINK?

Liquids *can* make you fat! They contain calories, and calories count.

Remember, 3,500 calories are equivalent to one pound of
body weight (fat), and each of the following contain 3,500
calories:
- 14 White Russians
- 20 cans of regular beer
- 24 cans of cola
- 36 glasses of wine
- 40 cans of light beer

The caloric contents of popular beverages are listed in
Table 11.1.

THE ART OF DRINKING

Thirst can be worse than hunger. Our urge to drink is often
stronger than our need for food. Drinking can cause two
problems: (1) Weight gain—due to the calories in the drinks
and (2) Impaired physical and mental performance.

It is important to reduce these problems to a minimum or to
eliminate them completely. The tricks to achieve this are

Table 11.1
Caloric Content of Different Beverages

Drink	Quantity	Calories
Nonalcoholic		
Coffee or tea	1 cup	2
Orange juice	1 glass (6 oz)	20
Chocolate milk	1 glass (8 oz)	215
Cola	1 can (12 oz)	140
Other sodas	1 can (12 oz)	140–160
Diet sodas	1 can (12 oz)	1 or 2
Alcoholic		
Beer, regular	1 can (12 oz)	160–180
Beer, light	1 can (12 oz)	70–110
Liqueurs	1 jigger	150–200
Gin; Rum	1 jigger	110
Whiskey, Vodka	1 jigger	110–120
Mixed drinks w/sugar	1 glass (8 oz)	160–300
Wine, white or rosé	1 glass	100
Wine, red	1 glass	160

easy. However, in accordance with our line of thinking, let's get to know the enemy first.

Drinking Alcoholic Beverages

The calories in alcoholic drinks come from the alcohol itself and from the added sugar. This is a real problem because the alcohol and the sugar increase each other's actions. There have been several studies that demonstrated that there is an initial "high" after the consumption of sweetened alcoholic beverages, which lasts about one to one and a half hours, followed by a "low," which causes a person to be tired, sleepy, aggressive, and depressed. These effects are especially serious if the consumption of these drinks occurs on an empty stomach.

The following is the typical pattern of the causes and effect of low blood-sugar levels: Sugar ends up in the bloodstream and we get a false "high," which is increased by the intoxicating effect of alcohol. The pancreas then reacts, releasing insulin. The alcohol starts to wear off, and the blood-sugar level drops rapidly. If this happens before dinner, we try to compensate by overeating.

Shakespeare once said of alcohol, "It provokes the desire, but takes away the performance." Many good books have been written about drinking and alcohol consumption, and most of us know how it affects our bodies and our minds, so we will skip a detailed discussion.

Alcohol is of interest to the gerontologist for two reasons: 1. Longevity studies have shown that drinking one to two alcoholic beverages per day increases life spans. This depends somewhat on body weight and physical activity. This also agrees with my own theory on health: We don't have to become fanatics in order to live a healthier and longer life.

2. When alcohol is broken down or metabolized, aldehydes are formed. According to several theories, these aldehydes have been blamed for forming free radicals, the bullets that actually cause aging. The aldehyde intermediates are also believed to destroy vitamin A, which is needed to metabolize alcohol in the liver. Alcohol metabolism also requires more B vitamins; some experts in this field have stated that alcohol depletes B vitamins.

Since we know that alcohol consumption increases our need for B vitamins and for additional antioxidants such as vitamins A, E, and C and for the trace mineral selenium, now, we want to mention a few rules that will eliminate most problems.

THE DIETERS' RULES ON DRINKING AND QUENCHING THIRST

1. Try not to drink on an empty stomach. If you do, never drink sweetened drinks; they will play havoc with your blood sugar.

2. Whenever you are thirsty, quench your thirst with an alcohol-free, low-calorie drink.

You should know the caloric content of drinks. Mixed drinks, especially the ones with sugar, often push a dieter's caloric intake over the limit. Also, these drinks cause more problems if your weight loss is hampered by a special insulin sensitivity.

Remember the noncaloric mixers: club soda, seltzer, mineral water, plain water, and noncaloric healthy fizzes like Vita-Fizz from Nutrition Science Laboratories or "Emergen-C" from Alacer Company. Use them to dilute your other drinks. A wine spritzer (wine and club soda) contains only about 45 calories if made with these mixers. Most regular sodas are far too sweet; you can cut their calories by more than 50 percent by diluting them with plain soda water.

Coffee and tea, without sugar, have only about one calorie per cup. Diet drinks are preferred because they have almost zero calories, but the saccharin is still a risk factor that shouldn't be ignored.

For the duration of your weight-loss program, try to stay away from sugar-sweetened liqueurs. These drinks are extremely high in calories, and as you saw in chapter 10, the sugar might completely prevent your body from burning fat.

12

FOOD ALLERGIES: How they can make you crave certain foods.

> All ailments, except those resulting from birth defects, infection, or accident, have a common denominator, and that is foods and our chemical reactions to them.
>
> Mark Lovendale, M.D.
> Director, Medical Service Center
> Irvine, CA

CHECK YOURSELF

Food allergies can cause addictions and strong cravings for foods; this often happens with the processed junk foods that we should avoid. For example, if you are allergic to ice cream, it becomes very difficult to control the intake of this "food." Therefore, it is important to find out if you are allergic to any foods.

1. Do you know if you are allergic to any foods? YES NO
2. Did you ever have your allergies checked by either skin or cytotoxic tests? YES NO
3. Did you ever go on the four-day rotation diet? YES NO

If you answered "YES" to at least items 1 and 2 or 1 and 3—and if you are already taking the right action—you can move on to the next chapter.

THE BASIC ADDICTION IDEA

If you are allergic to a food (usually a "bad" food), you will become addicted and crave this food, making it more difficult for you to avoid it. Why does this occur?

When you eat a food that you are allergic to, your body goes into overdrive and tries to adapt to this "wrong" food; this gives you an "up" feeling. If this happens frequently, the "up" feeling won't happen anymore, and the only thing that will result is the stress that remains as your body attempts to deal with the nutritional insult; the overall result will be a "down" feeling. It's like beating a horse that's already too tired from too much running. It's asking your body to deal with an additional insult when it hasn't recovered from the last one yet; thus, you become addicted to foods from which you expect an "up" but that, in reality, produce a "down."

Let's compare this to cigarette smoking, which is one of the most common addictions. The first time people smoke, they don't "come alive with pleasure" as the happy smokers in the ads do. The smokers usually feel dizzy and sick to the stomach. That's the first time. If they decide to continue, the second time is easier and by the tenth time it's a snap. What has happened is that the body adapted to the poisons in the cigarette smoke, and a reaction that scientists call the "adaptation response" has gone into effect. Adaptation leads to addiction. The "pickup" smokers get from cigarettes is caused by the specific adaptation response; the body goes into overdrive to deal with the poison. As time goes by the adaptation stops and so does the pickup. The smokers suffer with nervousness, depression, or headaches (the withdrawal symptoms of a cigarette addict), and they have an instinctive, driving urge to feel good again (hence, the craving for another cigarette). They're hooked.

You can also be addicted to food. Bear in mind that food

addiction is an allergy and many people become allergic to the substances they are most exposed to such as sugar, junk foods, or pollen. Pollen can cause a stuffy nose, wheezing, plus breathing problems. With food allergies, the body may cope with them by gearing up a specific adaptation response; a craving for the lift from the foods it's allergic to. If someone with food allergies doesn't eat those foods, withdrawal symptoms occur. If the person eats those foods frequently, the body is forced into the adaptation response too often, and it is put under extreme stress. Before the body can recover from going into overdrive, it is forced into doing it again. More stress and exhaustion result. It's like a boxer who gets hit, then gets hit again before he can recover from the previous blow.

ALLERGIES CAN PLAY A KEY ROLE IN WEIGHT CONTROL

If a person is allergic to a food that is consumed often, the resulting fluid retention can actually bring about a weight gain and make weight loss very difficult.

Chuck Coker, Olympic trainer and physical fitness expert, described a typical case. "A banker in our club was slightly overweight. He weighed 175 pounds, had a small potbelly and had a roll around his middle. He ran six miles a day and worked out three times a week in the weight room. He was constantly constipated, so his doctor had prescribed bran every morning to provide him with relief. I suspected he was allergic to wheat and suggested that he have a cytotoxic test performed, Out of 160 food substances, he was allergic to 42, including wheat. After two months on a diet that eliminated the foods he was allergic to, he was down to 150 pounds. He looked younger, felt terrific, and had an abundance of energy and no more headaches. He said he would never go back to his old life-style because he felt so good."

TESTING FOR FOOD ALLERGIES

There are basically three methods to check for food allergies. The last one you can practice yourself and does not require a visit to the doctor.

Skin Tests

The professional can tell how allergic you are to different concentrations of food extracts scratched or injected under the skin, by measuring the degree of the reaction. This method is somewhat time-consuming and is becoming outdated.

Cytotoxic Tests

A doctor draws a small sample of your blood; it is shipped to a laboratory where the actual tests are done. Samples of food extracts are mixed with your blood and the reaction is observed under the microscope. How allergic you are to any one of the approximate 150 foods tested is expressed on a scale of 0 to 4. This method is excellent but somewhat expensive (the test costs from three hundred dollars to four hundred dollars). The earlier cytotoxic tests were not very precise and reproducibility was questionable. However, most laboratories have changed the testing procedure and some now call it hypersensitivity testing. If done by a good laboratory, the results are quite reliable.

The GAMA Assay, a test that is more precise, is being developed by Dr. Richard Wright (formerly at UCLA) of Physicians Laboratory in Los Angeles. This is a relatively new test, and only a small number of doctors are using it. So, if you want to have this done, you might have to make a few phone calls to holistic- and/or prevention-oriented doctors.

The Four-Day Rotation Diet

The rules are simple. You are allowed to eat any food only once every four days. In this way, you will learn to recognize any food allergies, and your body has time to recover if an allergic reaction occurs.

You can recognize an allergic reaction by an increase in your temperature, as if you had a slight cold; also, your sinuses might puff up, or you might feel as if something is not quite right. If this happens, watch for a reaction when you expose yourself to this food again. There can be weak reactions, and there can be strong ones that make you feel itchy all over. Besides helping you recognize the foods you are allergic to, this diet will also help you feel better because you are not subjected to the same food allergens at all times. The more allergic you are to a specific food, the more you should avoid it. But don't avoid it totally. By subjecting your body to those foods from time to time, it might learn how to deal with those "poisons."

If you are allergic to a number of foods, you must avoid them because they can cause the retention of fluids, affect your mood, and reduce your energy level. Whether you do it "cold turkey" or slowly simply depends on you. If you have some withdrawal symptoms, just keep at it and use a little willpower.

People who are allergic to food usually know it; we really only want to call your attention to the fact that allergies *can* be an obstacle in your weight-loss program.

If you crave any specific foods, including sweets, then you should pay attention to this topic and at least follow the four-day rotation diet.

What we have outlined here will be sufficient for most people to determine if they should use any follow-up procedures. A more detailed, nutritional, approach to allergies is outlined in the *Supernutrition Handbook.* (See Appendix D.)

One of the best summary papers dealing with Chemical Hypersensitivity, written by Drs. Stephen Levine and Jeffrey Reinhardt, was just recently published in the *Journal of Orthomolecular Psychiatry.* An excellent newsletter, the *Allergy Research Review,* is published by Nutri-Colony of Concord, California.

13

UNSTABLE APPETITE: Eating disorders require a rearrangement of weight-loss priorities.

> There are eating disorders and disorders caused by eating the wrong foods. Binging and bulimia are just two of those self-induced disorders.
> Robert Mendelsohn, M.D.
> Author of *Male Practice*

Susan. K. "This is depressing. If I wasn't a Catholic, I'd kill myself. I wonder if I could really do it since I don't seem to be able to do anything right. I tried this new low-cal diet and I exercised on top of it. In three days I was able to lose four pounds. I was like on a high and thought that maybe this time it will work. I don't even know how it happened, but I just wanted to scream when I found myself in a corner of our cafeteria, gulping down everything there was on display. I cried and cursed when I tried to throw it all up again in the bathroom. I am 20 pounds overweight and this habit I got myself into is tearing me apart."

The above is a direct quote from a 32-year-old woman who came to see us about her eating disorder: bulimia. Once a week she came to a counseling session in which she learned everything about what we now call "The Holistic Medicine Approach to Binging and Bulimia." Within six weeks she reduced her binge-purge habit from an average of three to four times per week to just once every two weeks. After seventeen weeks she was no longer bulimic, and she had also lost thirty pounds. Our approach will be summarized at the end of this chapter.

Our work with people who suffer from binging or bulimia made one thing crystal clear: If you have an eating disorder, you *must* emphasize a number of key weight-loss factors in order to shed the desired weight and/or eliminate your disorder. Your priorities, due to the eating disorder, might be quite different than what we might suggest for any other person. Not dealing with this problem correctly could make your weight-loss program a total failure.

Therefore, in this short discussion, we want to find out if you have an eating disorder, and if so, we want to tell you what has worked for our patients and how to rearrange your priorities to achieve your desired goal. If, after reading about the following eating disorders, you find that one of them applies to you, then reading this chapter and reevaluating your weight-loss priorities is a must.

ANOREXIA NERVOSA

This eating disorder involves an obsession with thinness and a chronic lack of appetite, induced by complex emotional disorders.

Some obvious symptoms are excessive weight loss, the absence of menstruation (a sign of below-average body fat), moodiness, and social isolation; less noticeable symptoms are feelings of loneliness, inadequacy, insecurity, and stress. Food intake, when calculated as outlined in chapter 3, is usually far below what it should be.

Some time ago, an extremely skinny young woman consulted with me about her problem. She ate almost nothing for breakfast and lunch. When her boyfriend took her out for dinner, she would self-induce vomiting immediately after the meal because she was so afraid the food would make her fat. She was classified as anorexic bulimic.

If you suffer from anorexia, this book is not for you; the only thing it might teach you is to eat sufficient amounts of foods. Don't attempt to lose any weight, and do seek professional help; you may be in danger. The death of the singer Karen Carpenter was not an isolated case; it is estimated that from 5 percent to 10 percent of all anorexics die from disorders associated with malnutrition.

BINGING

This eating disorder involves excessive sporadic consumption of large amounts of foods, very often sweets. As a result, there is often a weight gain. Many bingers then feel so guilty about having eaten so much that they starve themselves for long periods of time.

From a holistic point of view, dealing with the binger is relatively easy *if* the person is willing to take advice and really wants to do something about the problem.

BULIMIA, THE BINGE-PURGE SYNDROME

Essentially the bulimic is a binger with an additional problem. Often, after unsuccessful attempts to deal with food intake or a weight problem, the bulimic learns how to induce vomiting. Bulimia is far more prevalent than anorexia. Estimates suggest that 15 percent to 20 percent of all women with above-average intelligence are practicing bulimia; just recently, Jane Fonda revealed that she had been a bulimic for more than twenty years.

"What an easy way to control your weight problem. All you do is go to the bathroom, stick your finger down your throat, and all caloric problems are flushed down the toilet. And soon you start to wonder why you don't lose any weight. You come to the conclusion that there is something seriously wrong with your metabolism," said one of my now-recovered bulimics, when she was recalling her first year of binge purging.

As an alternative to purging, bulimics often use other means, such as ingesting excessive amounts of laxatives, to prevent the absorption of foods.

The symptoms for bingers and bulimics are very much the same: moodiness, depression, low self-esteem, and being a perfectionist often go together. Bingers and bulimics are always fighting with those few extra pounds. They read one diet book after another and fail to see the major problem, namely, that their habits actually induce a loss of lean muscle mass. Because bulimics are depressed, they tend to look older, once the problem is overcome, they have a new lease on life and the improvement becomes outwardly visible.

The foods consumed by the bulimic are mainly sweets and fat foods, and what is often a paradox is the fact that when they practice binge purging, they have less control over their weight than during the time they carefully watch what they eat.

The anorexic, binger, and bulimic should understand that these disorders are all curable. Professionals in this field are developing new approaches that are very successful. For a number of years we have been working with bingers and bulimics and our success rate is extremely good. We get a 60 percent to 70 percent success rate after about four months of counseling, whereas eating-disorder clinics claim the same success rate after about one year of counseling.

THE ORTHODOX VERSUS THE HOLISTIC-MEDICINE APPROACH

Bulimia was recognized as a disorder as late as 1980, when it was entered in the diagnostic *Statistical Manual of Mental Disorders*. This means that bulimia is classified as a mental disorder.

Few professionals in holistic and preventive medicine would agree with this definition; most of these professionals believe that bulimia is a self-induced disorder, caused by eating the wrong foods and practicing the wrong health habits, with underlying psychological problems.

Let's look at the three basic approaches in treating bulimia.

1. *Psychology and psychiatry.* In these fields bulimia is generally treated as a mental disorder. The psychologists and psychiatrists look at the bulimics and say that these people are mentally ill and that's why they binge and purge. There are lots of psychologists and psychiatrists who treat this eating disorder but they know nothing about nutrition; their nutritional advice is often superficial. They often test their patients and find that they suffer from depression; then, they treat the depression with drugs that can lead to other problems and can have horrendous side effects. They feel that the patients will go back to eating "normally" when their mental disorder is cured. They don't acknowledge the fact that almost 100 percent of bulimics don't know what "eating normally" is. Except for a few knowledgeable nutrition-oriented professionals, they don't take into account that eating the wrong foods can induce eating disorders.

2. *Eating-disorder clinics.* Here they recognize that bulimia is a problem that has a lot to do with the patient's food intake. Medical tests include depression scores that are usually high, meaning that clinical depression is established. The nutrition counseling is very basic and, in the eyes of the nutrition-oriented professional, insufficient. They talk about the four basic food groups. They try to make the patient aware of the fact that, in general, eating lots of sweets and junk food is not good nutrition.

Their methods are a slight improvement over the ones used by psychologists and psychiatrists because some direct nutrition counseling is included. However, in their approach, they also often treat the depression with drugs.

From a preventive medicine point of view, the approach of the eating-disorder clinics is also unsatisfactory because it doesn't acknowledge the junk foods, sweets, and faulty health habits as a possible *cause* for depression and for self-induced hunger mechanisms.

3. *Holistic Medicine.* The basic thesis: Medical statistics clearly show that faulty health practices and faulty nutrition are contributing factors to the onset of disorders such as

atherosclerosis, diabetes, and depression, and that the right health practices and good nutrition can reverse these disorders. Why shouldn't this same principle apply to bulimia?

The holistic approach always evaluates the patient's nutrition with precise computer techniques. We consistently find that it is far from satisfactory. Other health practices, such as physical activity, are also below the minimum acceptable levels. Blood-sugar problems, from real to temporarily self-induced hypoglycemia, are found in 100% of our patients. In a survey of four hundred bulimics we have found that the absolute majority of them was brought up on junk foods, that parents rarely emphasized good nutrition and regular meal patterns, and that the girls were rarely encouraged to be physically active and to participate in sports. We also found that bulimics have a below-average amount of lean muscle mass; this is even true for bulimics who fall into normal weight ranges and/or who have an exercise program. Hair analysis data also show that many minerals are below acceptable ranges.

Despite the fact that bingers and bulimics have read an average of six to nine diet books each, we have yet to find one single person who understands and correctly practices the nutritional principles that we find so helpful in eliminating their problems.

A FEW MORE FACTS ABOUT HUNGER MECHANISMS

Sugar consumption can induce low blood-sugar levels and a craving for sweets. Starving yourself and skipping meals can induce a general hunger mechanism; a hunger mechanism that asks for fat foods. Stress can also induce hunger mechanisms.

In bingers and bulimics we often find several self-induced hunger mechanisms at the same time. When they learn how to prevent these hunger mechanisms, it immediately reduces the number of binge-purge occurrences. Teaching people how to deal with stress has the same effect. A good exercise program can reduce stress and fully eliminate depression; again, it reduces binge purging.

RECOMMENDED ACTIONS

The material presented here is neither a complete discussion of the binge-purge syndrome nor is it an established treatment for these disorders. In this book we are dealing with weight loss and, from our experience in working with bingers and bulimics, we can tell you what has worked well for our patients. Applying our recommendations won't do any harm, and they can definitely help in solving the problem.

If you have an eating disorder such as binging or bulimia, the following chapters and actions have a very high priority in our program. In addition, give high priority to the weight-loss factors in Figure 10.1 and in the anti-aging weight-loss checklist (Fig. 17.1).

Chapter 3
Learn to balance your caloric act. Your caloric intake should never be far below your calculated caloric requirements. Weight loss must be steady and slow.

Chapter 5
Always eat regular meals. The meals can be small, but never skip a meal to save calories. Make sure that each meal contains at least some lean protein. Have very small amounts of a protein drink between meals.

Chapter 7
Start a good exercise program that includes exercise machines to build lean muscle mass. Never exercise without first eating breakfast or when you haven't eaten for a long time. Allow at least thirty minutes from the time you eat until you start exercising.

Chapter 8
Learn to handle distress. Read the recommended books. If

this doesn't do the trick, learn to meditate. Possibly take a stress-management class.

Chapter 9

If you can eliminate all sugar and sweets from your diet, success will be much easier to achieve. Sugar and sweets are a big temptation, but remember all the bad reactions they start in your body. Never have any kind of sweets on an empty stomach.

Chapter 4

Have plenty of "negative-calorie foods" in the refrigerator.

Earlier we mentioned that psychological factors are also a big part of the picture. You can deal with some of them (e.g., depression and stress) by taking the correct actions as outlined in the various chapters; but to deal with this aspect in more detail, we have included a number of booklets in our approach. Three booklets, entitled *Understanding and Overcoming Bulimia* are available from Gürze Books in Santa Barbara and are shipped in a plain envelope. (See Appendix D.)

Don't read all the booklets at the same time. Take them step by step. Start with any one of the booklets. Read it twice during the first week. During the second week read it again and *write* down (do not underline) what you found applicable to your personal situation. Review the basic message in the booklet.

By the third week you can read the second booklet. A few days later read it again. Allow yourself some time to do that. During the fourth week read it again and write down what you found applicable for yourself. and why it was applicable. In the fifth week you read the third booklet. Follow the same approach that you practiced for the other booklets.

Later, when you get to the anti-aging weight-loss checklist, make sure to check all the items every day. You will soon find connections between faulty nutrition, other health practices, and the frequency of the binge-purge occurrences; there will be fewer when you apply the health principles correctly, more when you are careless and don't pay attention.

As you continue this approach, you will truly learn how to take charge of your own health. If you find you still have problems, keep digging in and possibly ask a professional for help.

Remember, Rome wasn't built in one day.

Table 13.1

BULIMIA—HIGHLY SPECIFIC
HAIR ANALYSIS PATTERNS
(Research by Hans J. Kugler, Ph.D.)

Hair samples from twenty patients—all suffering from bulimia —were analyzed by Mineralab and Doctor's Data. All patients, females with ages from 18 through 47, showed the following hair analysis patterns:

CALCIUM and MAGNESIUM: extremely high despite the fact that their dietary intake of these minerals was at least 20 percent below the RDA. In patients who were able to normalize their eating patterns, and who included sufficient amounts of protein in their diets AND a calcium/magnesium supplement, hair analysis data slowly came down toward more normal values. It is believed that, before the dietary changes were implemented, these two minerals were not absorbed into the cells and therefore showed the high hair analysis values.

CHROMIUM: far below standard ranges. This mineral is very important for blood sugar homeostasis.

ZINC: slightly below standard ranges in 90 percent of the patients.

SELENIUM: very low in all patients. This mineral is extremely important for maintaining good immune functions.

SODIUM and POTASSIUM: far below reference ranges, but this was considered insignificant because these two minerals can be leached out of the hair due to frequent washing, blow drying, and other hair treatments.

OTHER MINERALS: even though often on the low side, showed no great variations or deviations from data obtained for the average population.

OTHER RECOMMENDED ACTIONS

1. Make an appointment with your doctor for a physical and a blood analysis. An eating disorder means that you may have many medical disorders. (Because of these disorders, you probably will be covered by your medical insurance.)

2. Have a hair analysis done to check the mineral status in your body. A lack of key minerals is often found in people with eating disorders; this can have serious consequences. If you can't get a hair analysis through your doctor, see Appendix D.

3. We use *The Weight and Appetite-Control Workbook* for our patients who suffer from eating disorders. It contains many principles that are outlined in this book, but there is lots of information about eating disorders, a detailed discussion of the holistic medicine thesis on binging and bulimia, and the results of a survey of bulimics. It is especially tailored for the bulimic. Again, see Appendix D for more details.

14

WEIGHT-LOSS MEASURES: The ones that failed the test.

> If people only knew how many medical problems can be induced by those diet and weight-loss gimmicks, they wouldn't even consider using them.
>
> David Wong, M.D.
> Director, Health Integration Center
> Torrance, CA

When we ask people to take charge of their own lives, and ask them to contribute just a little effort to achieve what they want, there are always a few who are very willing to abandon the plan and take some unproven and often totally idiotic shortcuts. These are the true masochists! They don't really want to succeed; they thrive on their misery.

On the off-chance that you might abandon our common-sense approach and attempt one of those weight-loss "miracles" that are eventually always proven wrong, let's take a look at a few more facts and weight-loss fallacies.

INTESTINAL BYPASSES AND STOMACH STAPLING

Modern medicine often comes up with some truly lunatic advice. In my opinion, stomach stapling and digestive tract bypasses belong under this heading.

In order to reduce food intake and/or food absorption, a small number of people have undergone surgery in which the stomach is literally stapled to make it smaller, or, in another procedure, a part of the digestive tract is bypassed and food now moves through the body faster, without being completely absorbed.

Can you imagine that some people would rather subject themselves to the knife of a surgeon instead of practicing some simple self-discipline and good nutrition? The pain of surgery is not the only consideration; resulting scars are also painful and reduce a person's ability to do urgently needed physical exercises. Also for quite some time, any sexual activity is impossible or greatly restricted.

Their mood changes, and what their bodies don't absorb doesn't get to their cells. Gastrointestinal disturbances, diarrhea, and so forth, are frequently side effects. Important vitamins and minerals wind up in the toilet instead of in your internal organs.

During several meetings, doctors have commented on these procedures, and it has become quite clear that intestinal bypass surgery performed on extremely obese patients to help them lose weight causes more harm than good and should not be done. Drs. Charles Clayman and Daniel O'Reilly of Northwestern University, in an editorial in the *Journal of the American Medical Association*, said that intestinal bypass surgery was metabolically and physiologically unsafe. Many prevention-oriented doctors would certainly agree with these researchers. There are, however, other doctors who still practice bypass surgery. Most people believe that bypass surgery is only done as a last resort. This is not so. Many doctors are still very knife happy.

How effective is it? Good statistical data are not available. However, I can tell you about a friend who had bypass surgery when he was a hundred pounds overweight. He lost the weight after the surgery, but he really felt miserable. He was depressed and no longer an aggressive businessman. Then he developed kidney stones. After this problem was remedied, he had his bypass reconnected and went through more expenses, more pain, and more depression. He also started to regain weight. Then he came to see me and learned how to eat right, exercise, and watch those calories. He now has his weight problem under control.

Stomach stapling to reduce the size of the stomach and to reduce total food intake appears to fail even more. Instead of eating three large meals, people who have had the stapling surgery done now eat five to ten small meals per day, and many of them are still overweight.

Many of the risks associated with this type of surgery were discussed in a paper by Dr. H. Buchwald and others, entitled "Searching for the Best Weight Reduction Operation," and published in *Surgery*. Keep in mind that a nonsurgical approach, using exercise and caloric restrictions can be successful even for grossly obese patients, as reported by Dr. R. Lapman.

SPOT-REDUCING

No matter if you use special exercises, suits, or belts that make you sweat, or those magic creams, spot-reducing doesn't work; scientific proof was published by Dr. Frank Katch in a number of journals. Excess sweating can be harmful by causing skin rashes or by causing mineral losses from your body.

Weight loss always occurs evenly on your body, no matter what you do to specific parts of your body. The only way to shape your body is by combining weight loss with exercises that build specific muscle groups.

HOW ABOUT "DREAMING YOUR FAT AWAY"?

Do you really believe that taking a few pills before bedtime can make your fat disappear? What could possibly happen in your dreams to produce this weight loss? Would you really spend money for such a product?

Could there be a scientific basis for these new pills? The pills contain two amino acids, ornithine and arginine, in the 100-milligram range. Research on animals shows that very large amounts of arginine and ornithine can stimulate the pituitary to release growth hormones into the bloodstream. Since growth hormones stimulate muscle growth, metabolism should be increased.

Ornithine and arginine are not new substances; they are amino acids found in every protein. Taking small amounts, as contained in these tablets, will do absolutely nothing to stimulate your pituitary. In order to possibly get some pituitary stimulation, you would have to take at least 6 grams of ornithine or 12 grams of arginine, and preferably on an empty stomach.

Not one single study on humans has demonstrated that taking such large quantities of these amino acids is safe. People who have tried large amounts tell us that nausea is a major problem, and most of them quit before seeing any results.

Bodybuilders are always looking for a new method to increase muscle mass. In 1983 a large number of the members of some health clubs decided to try these amino acids. I gave them my address and told them to let me know if they got good results. I received only negative reports.

What is more important though is the fact that a major health risk has been established. Arginine increases the risk of herpes. The herpes virus needs arginine to grow and duplicate.

Any real results with these amino acid combinations would be only very minor and would definitely have to be combined with other weight-loss action.

AMYLASE INHIBITORS—STARCH BLOCKERS

Just a short time ago there were several new products on the market, which contained a material that inhibits the hydrolysis of starchy foods. This material is a natural product, often made from a special type of bean. At first glance it may sound good. All we have to do is swallow a little pill that contains no artificial ingredients and that prevents the complex carbohydrates from hydrolyzing and converting into sugar. Up to 50 percent of all calories in some meals are carbohydrates that won't be absorbed.

In our earlier discussion of nutrition (chapters 3 and 4), we pointed out that these complex carbohydrates are the carbohydrates that are good for you because they hydrolyze (change) into glucose very slowly. This is desirable in order to maintain normal blood-sugar levels.

If you take an amylase inhibitor and the complex carbohydrates are not digested, then only the simple sugars in the foods get into the bloodstream. This is comparable to eating a meal that consists only of protein, fats, and sugar. If you don't include any sugar with such meals—which is not recommended anyway—the body now has to use fat to get energy. This causes the formation of ketone bodies (chemicals that change the pH in the body, that make you urinate frequently, and that throw a monkey wrench into many normal processes in your body). We are back to the diet idiocies of protein and fat only. In essence, this type of diet induces the symptoms of diabetes.

There is another problem associated with these products: The body becomes more susceptible to blood-sugar changes; it acquires the ups and downs associated with sugar consumption, and lean muscle mass is broken down to keep blood-sugar levels normal. This lean muscle mass is extremely important in order to maintain normal blood-sugar levels. Therefore, starch blockers have been removed from sale in most states; however, you will often find someone who'll sell you a miracle pill no matter what.

The only possible way to use starch blockers correctly (assuming that they have no other druglike side effects) is to use them in combination with a high-starch diet that is also low in refined sugars and fats. In essence, a low-fat Italian meal. Also, starch blockers could only be used in limited quantities in order to allow the hydrolysis of some of the complex carbohydrates. Vitamin and mineral supplementation would also be very important under these conditions.

You can have the same benefits, without the risks, by following the nutrition rules outlined in this book.

TEFLON-TYPE GASTROINTESTINAL-TRACT COATINGS

A number of synthetic fluids that are not absorbed by the body at all have been found to coat the lining of the digestive tract and prevent the absorption of almost all foods, including the important nutrients in the foods. These fluids contain very large polymeric molecules. Also, long-term effects of these polymeric coating fluids have not been fully researched. Biochemistry courses teach us that large molecules have to be hydrolyzed in order to be absorbed. However, as research with other polymeric molecules (e.g., dishwashing detergents) has demonstrated, small amounts can pass through the digestive tract inside the body. It was shown that dishwashing fluids usually end up in the liver, cause "fatty liver," and can cause malfunctions in this important organ. Since the liver is the most important detoxifying organ in the body, a fatty liver can be very harmful to your health. This is why, when you wash dishes, many health professionals are recommending the use of natural dishwashing fluids, available in your health-food store.

BEHAVIORAL THERAPY VERSUS DRUG THERAPY

Many people would like to believe that it's easier to just swallow a diet drug without making any sacrifices or any effort to learn right from wrong. Hundreds of drugs have been tried on test animals, but none has been shown to be safe and effective at the same time. There are a number of new diet drugs, being researched right now, that have a good chance of making it on the U.S. market. We have looked at many of them and we feel that not one is worth trying.

With each of them, there is always something that increases a disease risk and/or that accelerates the overall rate of aging. Unless such new drugs are proven 100 percent safe—which many professionals feel they never will be—we should stick to the proven approach outlined in this book.

In essence, our approach, is behavioral therapy—combining health practices to make life better.

At Pennsylvania State University, Dr. Linda Craighead and colleagues followed 120 women who practiced different approaches for their weight problems; in essence they either took diet drugs or else they used behavioral therapy. The behavioral therapy consisted of teaching people how to eat right, exercise, and so forth.

Even though, initially, the women in the diet-drug treatment groups lost more weight than those who practiced behavioral therapy, one year later, a follow-up showed a striking reversal in the relative efficiency of the various treatments. Women who took the appetite-suppressant drugs had regained 63 percent of the weight whereas the ones who practiced behavioral therapy regained only 17 percent of the weight they had lost. The researchers concluded that behavioral therapy is still the choice treatment.

How does all this fit into our anti-aging approach? Although drugs always have side effects that increase disease risks and many new diet-regimens increase premature aging, only good things are being discovered about our common-sense anti-aging approach.

Part 3

DOING IT RIGHT, WITH SUCCESS AND EASE

None are so old as those who live without enthusiasm.

Wayne Spence, M.D.

15

REWARDS FOR ATTAINING YOUR WEIGHT LOSS. How they keep you on the right track.

Back in college, as an art major, I always wanted to go to Europe, but never had the money to do so. Later when I had the money something wasn't right. I guess I felt that those European men wouldn't react so enthusiastically toward a slightly plump woman. But, oh boy, I really wanted to encounter the men! So I promised myself a trip to Europe as my reward for shedding fifteen pounds and for getting into shape. Once I had pictures of Europe in my mind, I couldn't get to my health club fast enough. I lost the weight more than two weeks prior to my departure date.

Was it worth the effort? You bet it was! I never enjoyed a reward more.

One of my weight-loss patients

Why do we do things? Most people work because they need the money to live. A paycheck is their reward. Lucky are the people who like their work, who truly enjoy it. They get paid for having fun.

Professional athletes train because they want to be top performers in their sports and achieving their goal is reward enough for most of them; monetary rewards naturally sweeten the deal and make them forget some of the pain that was required to get there.

Body shaping, done with specific exercises and training equipment, ranges from bodybuilding to increasing a bustline or reducing the size of a belly. The reward is an improved appearance.

Your goal is a desired weight loss. If you follow our approach, your reward will be a more appealing figure and a more youthful and healthy appearance. But there are many other rewards. You should know what they are. They will serve as positive reinforcements so that you don't quit when it gets a little difficult.

REWARDS, REWARDS; HELP IS ON THE WAY

By dividing the number of pounds you want to lose by three (for a small person) or by four (for a larger person), you will have an approximate idea of how many weeks it will take you to achieve your goal. Some people might lose weight a little bit faster, but remember not to overdo it.

While you are getting there, partial success will be a reward in itself, and it will prove to you that it can be done. You can give yourself additional support by learning about all other good changes that will take place. For example, you can add years to your life. Being overweight shortens your life span by six to twelve years. It doesn't cut six to twelve years off the end of your life, but it gets you there faster and condenses your entire aging cycle.

You want to achieve a normal weight because of the following:

- Excess pounds increase your risk of having a heart attack or stroke by more than 1,000 percent.
- Statistics tell us that nine out of ten diabetics were overweight when they were diagnosed as diabetics.

- Being overweight is associated with an increase in cancer. For overweight women, the onset of cancer of the breasts and ovaries is significantly higher.
- For men, a significant decrease in sexual functioning and hormonal imbalances is observed if the degree of being overweight is excessive.
- Being overweight makes you much more susceptible to depression and neurotic behavior.
- Being overweight reduces your body's own defense mechanism: the immune system. A decrease in immune functions has been associated with an increase in literally all other diseases and with an increase in the overall rate of aging.
- By following our program and without taking any risky shortcuts, you will be achieving body shaping at the same time, which will enable you to have the figure you have always wanted.

Evaluating all these points with your logical mind now makes it crystal clear that shedding those pounds—losing unneeded fat—is an absolute must. *You can do it!*

Don't give yourself any excuses!

You know that you can do it.

MORE POSITIVE REINFORCEMENT TO GET YOU THERE

I will share a secret with you. I, myself, have a real weight problem. If I don't carefully watch what I eat, don't get my exercise, or if I splurge just a little bit too much with drinks or desserts, I put on weight faster than I can count my calories. So I discipline myself with food and exercise, but I also follow several of the recommendations we discuss in the following chapters.

In my house, I post signs that reinforce my approach. On my refrigerator door, there is a sign that says, "Poor calorie counters acquire the figures to prove it." I used to have other signs all around the house, but since I've overcome my weight problem, I gave them away.

The Spenco Medical Corporation, located in Waco, Texas, has a great collection of educational and supportive posters and free catalogues. (See Appendix D.)

The posters are well designed and they deliver a clear message.

"FAT, the density that shapes our ends."

"BLUBBER feels just like it sounds."

"GLUTTONS are made, not born."

Other posters, also available in many good bookstores, deal with exercise, laziness, and general health.

REWARD YOURSELF

Set a goal for yourself: When you achieve your goal, give yourself a reward. Plan it well, and far enough ahead of time, so that you have something to look forward to.

A woman whom I counseled decided not to buy any clothes until she had reached her goal. She figured that she spent a certain amount of money per month on clothes. When she reached her desired weight, she went out on a shopping spree. The reward was twofold: Not only did she enjoy all her new clothes but her friends also noticed an entirely new person and complimented her.

A trip to a place you always wanted to visit . . .

A new car . . .

Anything . . .

Reward yourself!

A nosy reward

A woman who worked as a flight attendant for an airline consulted me about her weight problem, which was threatening to cost her her job. While we discussed nutrition and attempted to design a successful regimen for her, she happened to glance at a few pictures on my desk that showed the "before" and "after" of a nose job. Since her nose was just a little bit longer than average, she was very interested in the photos. I explained to her that one of the major signs of aging was a longer nose; as we grow older, the nose grows longer. A nose job, one of the simplest youth surgery operations, can make a person look ten to fifteen years younger. When we finished discussing her weight-loss program, she announced to me that after she reached her ideal weight, she would reward herself with a nose job.

It took her about two months to lose twenty pounds. During the second week of her weight-loss program, she consulted with a plastic surgeon and, subsequently, made a date for the nose job. She lost the weight, and she had the surgery, shaped up a little more, and bought new clothes. She truly was "a new woman." She told me: "It's like having the clock turned back twenty years."

What are you going to give yourself as a reward?

16

THEORIES ON AGING: How they confirm our advice and help you delay the signs of aging.

> Removing disease risk factors from your life will prevent aging as much as interfering with a true cause of aging. Preventing a disease means delaying aging to a great degree.
>
> Dr. Morton Walker
> Researcher and author of
> "The Bikini Diet."

Remember when we explained aging and getting older in chapter 1? We defined the rate of aging—how fast we get old—as a combination of at least one hundred different factors that either contribute to the onset of chronic diseases or to the true causes of aging.

We all know that there are many risk factors that contribute to, for example, heart disease. These are lack of exercise, faulty nutrition, a lack of certain vitamins, smoking cigarettes, to mention just a few. If we eliminate some of these risk factors, we will delay heart disease and our average life span will increase. The more diseases we can prevent, the longer our average life span will be. If we could totally prevent heart disease, the average life span might increase from the present 74 years to about 80 years. If we could prevent cancer and heart disease, the average life span might increase to 90 years; this is still quite a bit below the generally accepted maximum possible life span for humans: 110 to 120 years. If we were able to interfere with a true cause of aging, the entire aging process would be delayed, and the maximum life span might increase to a possible 120 to 130 years.

HOW DO WE TEST THEORIES ON AGING?

In our laboratory we used three different strains of mice. One type of mouse, the Snell Dwarf, has an average life span of only three to five months. This animal has an immune deficiency; if we can increase its life span, then we have done something about improving immune functions since, as you probably know, the immune system plays a key role in preventing disease.

The second type of mouse, a white mouse, is very similar to humans because it is cancer-prone, just as humans are. If we increase the life of these animals, then we have done something about improving immunity and preventing cancer. The third type of mouse is a mouse with a dark coat (the CB-57). This type and other similar types of mice don't die from specific diseases; they just get old and die. If we can increase the life span of this type of mouse, then we have done something about interfering with a true cause of aging. For the gerontologist, the last type of mouse is of the greatest interest.

Animal research suggests that it is already possible to interfere with the true causes of aging. However, the true causes of aging and the prevention of chronic diseases are closely connected. We find that people who have several disease risk factors in their life also look old earlier.

Most people are familiar with the fact that being overweight is a major risk factor for heart disease, diabetes, depression, and even cancer. However, certain factors—such as too much fat; foods containing cholesterol, and excess sugar; insufficient amounts of roughage; or lack of exercise— have also been directly or indirectly connected with these chronic diseases. Since any increase in a chronic disease is also an acceleration of the entire aging process, the importance of supernutrition and good health practices is confirmed.

DIFFERENT THEORIES ON AGING

In this chapter we will take a look at the most important theories on aging, explain them to you, and show you how they relate to and confirm the advice in this book. You will learn more about aging and how you can interfere with the true causes of aging in order to slow down your aging process. Since our approach also teaches you how to eliminate many disease risk factors, a partial reversal of aging and rejuvenation is definitely possible.

As you now read through these theories, keep in mind that the entire aging process is a combination of disease risk factors and the true causes of aging.

Metabolic-Products theory

One of the earliest theories of aging that evolved from a number of scientific research studies is the *metabolic products theory*. According to this theory, the accumulation of oxidation products in your body interferes with normal cellular reactions and causes aging.

As you go through a normal day and burn calories, oxidation products are formed, and when they accumulate in your body, you get tired. When you rest, the body's disposal system goes to work and eliminates those chemicals from your body. All this takes time, and that's why you need more sleep when you have worked especially hard the day before. If you don't allow yourself to rest long enough, your body is placed under stress and you have to start the next day with a body that hasn't yet come to its full equilibrium. The situation gets worse if you push your body to extremes and burn the candle at both ends and if you consume processed foods that have synthetic chemicals added to them and that are difficult for your body to excrete.

Gerontologists tell us that an average of seven to eight hours of sleep per night is most beneficial. More or less sleeping time gives a shorter life span. If a person sleeps excessively, this suggests that there is something wrong, the body is apparently trying to reach an equilibrium, but it never achieves the goal. We frequently find this in people with blood-sugar disorders. A blood analysis of people with blood-sugar problems often shows that their immune system is not working efficiently.

Diffusion theory

This theory looks at the body's capacity to excrete the oxidation products and calculates the rate of diffusion of the chemicals out of the cells so that they can be transported to the organs that excrete them. The most important conclusion we can draw from this theory is that it is important to supply our body with enough pure water, from six to ten glasses per day; this serves as a media to flush the oxidation products from the body.

Rate-of-living theory

This theory (first advanced in 1928) correlates the surface area of tissue with energy expenditure in different animals and humans. A connection was established between the metabolic rate and the life span of a species: The higher the metabolic rate, the shorter the life span, and vice versa. Thus, if we could lower the metabolic rate of a species, we should get an increase in the life span. However, our DCML would also be lower, and weight problems would be increased even further.

Theoretically, we can lower the metabolic rate if we lower the body temperature. This has been done on cold-blooded animals, such as fish. If fish are kept at slightly lower water temperatures, they live longer. However, for warm-blooded beings such as humans this can't be done. If we try to chill the bodies of warm-blooded animals, the metabolism increases to bring the body temperature back to normal. If we continue to chill the animals, things start to go wrong and the animals die. The only time our metabolism is slightly lower is at night when we sleep. We can help to lower the metabolism at night by sleeping in a cool room.

There are also some indications that vitamin E can help to lower the metabolism. We therefore want to take vitamin E at night and not in the morning. Since vitamin E works best in combination with selenium, take these two together in the evening. This suggestion also makes sense because vitamin C, which should not be taken together with selenium, is usually taken early in the morning.

During the day we want our metabolism to be high because a high metabolism means energy and because we need energy to perform work. A simple way to sometimes give our metabolism a push—and force the body to burn more calories—is to take a swim in a cold swimming pool or in the ocean. In California, where some people go swimming even in the winter when the ocean is somewhat cool, we used this factor in one of our weight-loss studies. We found that people who went for an early morning swim in the ocean burned up more calories and had fewer weight problems. People who live in colder climates also have a slightly longer life span.

These three theories also support the importance of a restricted caloric intake and staying slim and trim. A Cornell University experiment conducted by Dr. C. McCay achieved 60 percent life-span increases on test animals when these animals were fed a diet low in calories but high in quality. He also found that they had a below-average weight. Exercising is also supported by these theories because it increases the circulation and accelerates the excretion of oxidation products.

Free-radical theory

This theory has probably received the most support of all the theories on aging. It states that aging is due to the damaging effect of "free radicals" on living tissue. Free radicals are very reactive molecules or fractions of molecules that are formed mainly from oxidation products of foods under the influence of radiation or food additives or when the foods are not sufficiently protected by certain vitamins and minerals. The chemist's definition is that these free radicals carry a single electron. Since all other molecules have electron pairs, each time a free radical reacts with a molecule, it forms another radical. It's as if a bullet is creating another bullet in the process of damaging a target.

Cross-linked tissue has been found in a number of human organs, ranging from the brain to the aorta.

These free radicals, the bullets that can damage living tissue, can be deactivated with a group of compounds known as antioxidants. Vitamins E, C, and A and the trace mineral selenium are natural antioxidants. BHT and BHA are synthetic antioxidants. Life spans increased from 10 percent to 60 percent, for animals who were given antioxidant supplements, were achieved depending on the combinations and amounts of antioxidants used. These antioxidants also play a role in preventing cancer. Most recently, English researchers found a correlation between beta-carotene, a vitamin A precursor, in the blood and protection against several types of cancer.

Immunologic theory

This theory, researched extensively by Dr. Roy Walford, states that aging is due to decreasing immunologic functions. Our bodies' defense mechanisms are of the utmost importance, and when these functions diminish, we are left defenseless against even relatively harmless bacteria. This theory has received tremendous support from researchers in literally every area of health. Cancer, heart disease, and even mental disorders have been linked to insufficient immune functions. Life-span decreases have been associated with a number of factors, such as cigarette smoking, obesity, and distress, that can hamper immune functions. In 1984, a group of researchers demonstrated that distress greatly reduces immune functions, thus, connecting the *stress* (as discussed in chapter 8), and the *immunologic* theories on aging.

A well-functioning immune system is the key to the prevention (and often the treatment) of many diseases, from cancer and heart disease to aging. Many nutrients have been associated with increasing immune functions; they range from the A, C, E, and folic acid vitamins to minerals such as selenium, zinc, calcium, and magnesium.

All of these data support our vitamin and mineral supplementation recommendations. This theory also supports our recommendation to eliminate, or greatly reduce, the amount of sugar in the diet. Dr. E. Cheraskin of the University of Alabama School of Medicine, found that the activity of cells in the blood that belong to the immune system is reduced by more than 80 percent if increasing amounts of sugar are added to the diet. On the other hand, a high-quality diet, without sugar and low in fats, increases immune functions to peak performance.

In his book *Maximum Life Span*, Dr. Roy Walford emphasizes the importance of not being overweight and of using strong vitamin and mineral supplements. By combining these principles, he has achieved life-span increases of up to 20 percent in animals. This is an honest and well-documented book; it doesn't draw farfetched conclusions that indirectly promise you everything without any effort on your part.

In chapter 7, we mentioned DMG (dimethylglycine), a supplement that can give you more energy and stamina when you exercise. DMG also increases immune functions by activating high-energy phosphates in the body.

We can measure the immune status of a person by analyzing a number of variables in the blood; weight loss and an increase in physical activity usually show a drastic increase in immune functions.

Cell therapy theory

This method uses injections of cell preparations made from embrionic sheep tissues. This method was often regarded as a Frankenstein-type approach, but it recently gained scientific recognition when the use of radioactive tracers demonstrated that some of the basic principles were correct. Using cell injections made from thymus tissues it was also shown that immune functions could be greatly improved. In addition to this, the stunning results on Down's Syndrome children—normalizing their facial features and doubling their I.Q.s put this method into a completely new light.

DNA-damage theory

This theory is a combination of the thinking of several researchers in gerontology. Originally proposed by Dr. L. Szilard, it states that aging is due to an accumulation of damage to the DNA molecule. DNA is the basic large molecule in the nucleus of every cell that carries all the genetic information about the species. When damage repeatedly occurs and is carried over into new cells, the DNA becomes less efficient.

The body also has a DNA-repair mechanism that can restore the DNA to normal if all required conditions are fulfilled. To see if there were any connection between aging and the DNA-repair mechanism, researchers evaluated the efficiency of the DNA-repair mechanism in different species, and they found that there was a direct correlation between it and the maximum life span of a species. In order to facilitate repairs, we need building materials, and this is the point at which nutrition enters the picture. Natural unprocessed foods are high in nucleic acids. DNA is also a nucleic acid. The building blocks for all nucleic acids are the same; therefore, good nutrition can supply the building materials for the DNA-repair mechanism. Vegetables, whole-grain products, and fish are high in nucleic acids. Junk foods and highly processed foods are low in nucleic acids.

Damage to the DNA can occur through free radicals and the antioxidants again can prevent this damage.

All these findings support our advice about good nutrition and vitamin and mineral supplementation.

Death-hormone and limited-cell-replication theories

According to the death-hormone theory, the production of a death hormone is built into our genes and is released late in life. The limited-cell-replication theory is based on experiments by Dr. Leonard Hayflick, a professor at Stanford University. He found that human cells are capable of a limited number of cell divisions and that their potential to replicate decreases with age.

Both theories suggest that there is a limit to the human life span, and this would seem to be discouraging news to researchers in aging. But a closer look at the field of gerontology will demonstrate that there are virtually unlimited possibilities for the biochemist.

With regard to the theories just mentioned, Dr. Lester Packer, at the VA hospital in Martinez, California, demonstrated that the addition of vitamin E to cell cultures can actually double the number of cell divisions. Other compounds also look very promising. This evidence suggests that it is possible to interfere with a true cause of aging. Even if the number of cell divisions is limited, nothing indicates that we couldn't live for 100, 150, or even more, years.

Cybernetic theory

This theory, originally advanced by Dr. Still, suggests that aging is due to an increasing loss of control of the nervous system over all functions of the body. If there is a loss of control, it must be due to some kind of change in the nervous system, and that's where the most fascinating research in aging is now taking place.

The neuroendocrines, from the hypothalamus to the pituitary and the thyroid, trigger the release of many hormones that control the functioning of the body. An imbalance of certain chemicals, called neurotransmitters, in the neuroendocrines is a result of the aging process. What is so fascinating about it is that the normal balance of neurotransmitters can be restored with nutrients and certain natural compounds.

Combination theory

A result of my own longevity studies was published in the *American Laboratory* in 1974. It also focuses heavily on the balance of the neurotransmitters in the nervous system. Since the neurotransmitters are made by the body from amino acids, derived from protein, and since low blood-sugar levels can induce an imbalance of these neurotransmitters, our nutritional advice is supported again.

COMPARISON STUDIES

Often you will hear the argument that what applies to the test animals isn't necessarily true for humans. Therefore, let me explain how our longevity studies are done, and how they apply to humans.

For our longevity studies we use three groups of animals; the animals are cancer-prone, just as humans are. Group 1 is subjected to the mistakes many humans make. Their diet contains 20 percent sugar; they don't exercise, are subjected to cigarette smoke, drink regular tap water, and they don't receive any supplements.

Group 2 is the control. Everything is standard and average. No sugar is added to the diet, and they are not subjected to cigarette smoke. Exercise wheels are installed in their cages, but the animals are not forced to exercise; some of the animals use them for short time periods. Their drinking fluid is tap water, and they don't get any supplements.

Group 3 gets a number of supplements, ranging from general vitamins and minerals to antioxidants, DMG, and a few other life-extending factors that are under investigation. Naturally these animals are not subjected to cigarette smoke; they are forced to exercise in rotating drums; they are kept mentally active by frequently rearranging the equipment inside their cages; and they get a high-quality drinking water. Their basic diet is a high-protein animal chow.

The difference in life spans between group 1 and group 3 is close to 100 percent. The animals in group 3 are also leaner, and they show the obvious signs of aging (such as hair loss) much later than the animals in group 1.

These results overlap the data from studies of humans and can be seen from an evaluation of research performed by Prof. D. Breslow of the UCLA School of Public Health. Professor Breslow and his associates followed about seven thousand people for several years and looked at their nutrition and health practices in relation to average life spans. The factors these researchers evaluated were general nutrition, regular food intake, exercise, smoking, weight, rest, and stress.

Extrapolating their findings shows that people who made mistakes in all of these areas had an average life span of about 58 years. The average human life span—for people who do just a few things wrong—is about 73 years. The generally accepted maximum life span for humans is at least 110 to 120 years. Compare the 58-year-average life span for people who are doing things wrong to the maximum possible, and you again have a 100 percent difference.

We hope that all of this is proof for you that the best possible results are always achieved when you use a combination of factors, without leaving anything out. Even though a little bit more complex, this approach gives long-lasting and virtually risk-free results.

Let me emphasize again that this is not supposed to be a complete discussion of all anti-aging measures. That would be a book in itself. For further reading, I recommend *Maximum Life Span* by Dr. Roy Walford.

17

THE ANTI-AGING WEIGHT-LOSS CHECK-LIST: It can help make doing it foolproof.

> With this weight-loss checklist I lost the pounds faster than I could follow the instructions.
>
> Rita K.
> (one of our weight-loss candidates)

How does one win a war? By having the best army, navy, marines or air force? By taking advantage of a weather situation or a weakness in the enemy's defense? By having the best intelligence information about enemy movements and troop strength? By having the best group, company, or battalion leaders? By having the latest weapons systems or even a wonder weapon?

Not by a single one of the above!

Each single factor is important and can shift the balance of an individual battle (equivalent to losing a few quick pounds), but the entire war is won only if all of the factors are incorporated into the whole picture; there must be excellent planning, leaving nothing to chance.

What I am again saying is that the same approach is true for achieving your desired and lasting weight loss! We must include all the related weight-loss factors, establish how they are related, and then put it all together with good planning.

How can we make sure that all of this is taken into account correctly, that we are doing things right, that key factors are not neglected, and that the planning and strategy make sense? *By using a checklist.*

When I take my airplane out for some aerobatic flying, nothing can be left to chance. I want to make sure that everything, from the condition of the airplane to weather and standard procedures, is the way it should be. The checklist becomes a matter of life. Airline pilots use checklists covering hundreds of points. The checklists on the Columbia spaceflights are computerized and a flight is perfect only if nothing is overlooked; everything must check out A-OK.

We have designed a checklist (Fig. 17.1) for you to use in the *anti-aging weight-loss program* that will make the program foolproof.

To reach your weight-loss goal, we want to make sure that:

1. You don't overlook or accidentally forget a key factor.
2. You apply the weight-loss factors correctly.
3. You have a strategy that makes it possible to do what is necessary.

Knowing *what* you have to do and how to do it is very important, but the final proof for the success of a program only comes when you actually *do it.* That's why planning becomes so important. In my personal experience with weight-loss counseling, and from discussions with other professionals in this field, it becomes quite obvious that the lack of planning and strategy is what causes the failure of even good weight-loss programs.

Let me explain why this is so important. It is easy for me to tell you the minimum amount of exercises you should do, and it is easy for you to say that you are willing to do it, but what if you are so exhausted from your daily work that you just can't do it, or if you just don't have any time? What if any aspect of your weight-loss program takes so much out of you that it stresses a relationship. Or your performance at work suffers? It is easy for you to say that you are willing to pay attention to

Figure 17.1. The Anti-Aging Weight-Loss Checklist

Day: 1 2 3 4 5
 1.   Low metabolism indicated; physical
      activity stressed.
 2.   a. Weighed self in the mornings.
      b. Body measurements recorded.
 3.   a. Desired daily caloric intake
      b. Actual daily caloric intake
      c. Supernutrition guidelines followed
          (Tables 3.1–3.3).
 4.   a. High fiber emphasized.
      b. Low fat emphasized.
 5.   a. High-quality breakfast eaten.
      b. Small, quality lunch eaten.
      c. Dinner eaten before 7 P.M.
      d. Rich late-night snacks or drinks
          eliminated.
 6.   Vitamin and mineral supplements taken.
 7.   Correct exercise done.
 8.   a. Stress factors indentified;
          countermeasures evaluated.
      b. Daily activities and exercise well
          planned to reduce stress.
 9.   Possible blood-sugar problems indicated.
      a. Sugar and refined carbohydrates
          reduced.
      b. Physical activity stressed.
      c. Lean protein eaten in every meal.
      d. GTF supplement taken.
10.
11.
12.

all those important single factors, but what if you have a tendency to forget things? What if you simply forget to buy the right foods and then are stuck with the choice of eating nothing or of having some greasy junk food at a neighborhood fast-food stand? What if you forget to tell your friends that you are on a weight-loss program and they are planning a big evening with a culinary extravanganza for you?

What if . . . ? And what if . . . ?

The checklist is designed to make your weight-loss fool-proof and make planning easier for you. Take a quick look at the anti-aging weight-loss checklist. You'll find that it is very much like the anti-aging weight-loss profile (Fig. 10.1) but just a little bit more detailed and expanded as to how to do things.

We will now review the key items that play a role in your weight-loss program one more time in order to pinpoint what *you* have to do, and then, you can use the anti-aging weight-loss checklist at the end of every day to check if you did things right and to plan the next day.

YOU DON'T HAVE TO BE PERFECT

When we finish with the final review, you will have your perfect weight-loss program in front of you in the form of the completed anti-aging weight-loss checklist. If you were to apply all the recommended actions, you would probably lose too much weight. That's why we previously told you that you don't have to be perfect.

We also told you that each weight-loss action corresponds to a certain weight loss. In Table 17.1 we have summarized the major weight-loss actions, their daily caloric savings, and the equivalent weight loss per month. You might not like one or the other action. That's quite all right! Only do the absolute minimum and just combine the actions that apply to you for the desired weight loss. But be careful! Don't overdo it by pushing your weight loss past a safe limit. The more you push your weight loss to extremes, the higher your chance of damaging your health.

How long have you carried this extra weight around with you? Do you really think that it will make a big difference if you lose the weight in ten weeks instead of twelve weeks?

Before we review the items on your anti-aging weight-loss checklist, take a pencil and cross out all the points that you had checked "Doesn't apply" in Figure 10.1. This already reduces the checklist a little bit.

Also, in the following final discussion, read only about the items that were checked "Important to do" or "Not sure." If, after this final discussion, any "Not sure" checks still haven't been clarified, consider them unimportant for now or possibly use one of the computer programs (see Appendix D) to get an answer. Keep practicing the items you checked "Already doing."

If you wish, use a colored marker to differentiate between the actions you are already doing and the new ones that you had checked "Important to do."

THE ITEMS ON YOUR CHECKLIST

Item 1

Getting in tune with your body, and sensing how it reacts to how you treat it and feed it, is especially important for people with a weight problem. People who control their weight very well know exactly when to stop in respect to food intake and what to do if they have gone past their limit.

Assume that you are at a dinner party and you are being offered this delicious dessert that gets your taste buds going. Now you know that the extra 300 calories don't belong in your program, but always having to say "no" to yourself is no fun either. But you *do* have a choice. A person who understands the weight-loss principles knows that a 30 to 40 minute walk burns up about 300 calories. So, why not have the dessert and then take yourself and your date, spouse, dog, or kids for a walk. You can admire a sunset, observe Mother Nature, or watch the lights or action in a city. It really makes no difference at all where you go for a walk; I personally enjoy a walk on the beach in California as much as a stroll along the

Table 17.1
Actions and Pounds

Below are listed a number of weight-loss actions, their daily
caloric savings, and the equivalent in pounds per month. Since
these are average numbers, *your* results might be higher or lower,
depending on body weight and biochemical individuality.

Action	Average daily cal. savings	Equivalent pounds/month
1. Change from the average American diet (40% cal from fats, high in refined carbohydrates) to a diet slightly lower in fats (35%), refined carbohydrates reduced by about one-third, some vegetables and whole-grain products increased. Food volume consumed remains the same.	300	2.5
2. Change from the average American diet to a low-fat (25%–30% cal from fat), low-sugar (at least two-thirds of sugar removed) high–complex-carbohydrate diet. Food volume consumed remains the same.	700	6.0
3. Change from "no breakfast, irregular meals, late dinner" to regular eating patterns that always include breakfast and an early dinner.	100–200	1-2
4. Eliminate late-night high-		

cal snacks such as 3 cookies or 1 cup of ice cream or 2 beers or buttered popcorn, and change to low-cal, high-fiber snacks.	300–400	2.5–3.5
5. General 20% caloric reduction below the DCML. Example: If DCML is 1,750 cal/day, change to a daily caloric intake of 1,400 cal.	350	3.0
6. Change from a "no-exercise" life-style to a minimum-activity program that includes at least five 30-minute walks and a few other minor activities.	200	1.7
7. Change from a "no-exercise" life-style to an exercise program for best possible disease prevention (3 × per week, 30–40 minutes each, vigorous) plus a few long walks.	600–800	5–7
8. Enhance the average American diet that gives you less than the RDA in vitamins and minerals with a good supplementation program that includes B vitamins (estimated).	20–50	0.2–0.5
9. For people who have an extreme insulin sensitivity in which sugar blocks fat metabolism: Remove all sugars, even the ones hidden in foods.	increase in metabolism by 300–500 cal/day 2.5–4	

lakeshore in Chicago, or window-shopping along Fifth Avenue in New York or in Underground Atlanta.

Your metabolism is determined by your own biochemical individuality. No matter how fast or slow it is, don't complain about it—do something about it. You can increase it by building up your lean muscle mass; then count calories—nothing else works.

Item 2

You will agree by now that, in order to appreciate the success of your program, you must document the changes. Weight is a good indicator, but body measurements and body fat are often better.

If you are extremely overweight, measuring body fat isn't a high priority; it would only confirm that you should lose weight. However, it becomes important when you get close to your weight goal. Some people, especially when they finally find the way to shed weight successfully, have a tendency to go to extremes—they don't know when to stop. Knowing your body-fat percentage, and how it compares to healthy ranges, would tell you precisely when to stop. Please don't ignore these simple indicators of good health.

Item 3

In order to lose weight, your caloric intake must be less than what you burn up. *Nothing else works!* If somebody tells you that calories don't count, tell that person to go back to school. Sometimes somebody will tell you that it's the quality and type of foods that count. But when you add up the caloric content of the foods they recommend, you'll find that it's very low. So do yourself a favor and count calories.

Write down your desired daily caloric intake. Every day report what your actual daily caloric intake is by keeping a nutrition log (writing down everything you eat and drink) and adding up all the calories at the end of every day. Add up all the calories that were derived from fats and from proteins. Compare your actual food intake to our recommendations (Tables 3.1–3.3) and record if your nutrition was satisfactory.

Again, for most people it's not necessary to be perfect. Some people find themselves under extreme distress when they are asked to change their nutrition drastically. Tables 3.1–3.3 show you what your nutrition should be. In relation to what it actually is, improve it as much as you can to come closer to our recommendations. *Ease* into the program. You can always be a little bit stricter later.

Your nutrition will improve if you avoid fatty foods, make sure that the protein in your diet is from lean sources; eat lots of fresh, unprocessed (sometimes raw) vegetables and salad greens.

Item 4

Our nutrition guidelines in chapter 3 already included some lowering of fats, plus increasing high-fiber foods. For most people, this is satisfactory. However, if you really want to reduce your caloric intake but still feel hungry, you can further lower the fat content of your diet and increase high-fiber foods. There is absolutely nothing wrong with these adjustments, especially while on a weight-loss program.

Eating lots of "negative-calorie foods" can only improve your nutrition (chapter 4).

Item 5

Studies show that 90 percent of the people with weight problems skip meals and/or eat big dinners late at night. Need we say more? You learned the facts in chapter 5. If you dislike eating breakfast, at least have a protein drink. Any adjustment will make your weight loss easier. If you can't change from late to earlier dinners, then reduce the size of your dinner and the caloric content.

Item 6

We feel that the recommended vitamin and mineral supplements are *extremely important* for delaying aging and even for preventing cancer. These vitamins and minerals are included in the antiaging weight-loss program to ensure the best possible nutrition. However, they will have almost no effect on increasing or decreasing the degree of your weight loss. If your only concern is to lose a few pounds, if you are not interested in long-term health effects, if you only want to do the minimum, and if you don't like to take pills, then you can cut the vitamins from your weight-loss program. If you decide to do this, you can, to a certain degree, put your mind at ease by knowing that a change to the quality foods recommended will create some increase in your vitamin and mineral intake. The choice is yours.

For more good information about vitamin and mineral supplementation, read any one of the books by Drs. Emmanuel Cheraskin, Richard Kunin, Harold Rosenberg, or Richard Passwater.

Item 7

We have explained the importance of exercise repeatedly. You should know by now that a healthy weight loss is impossible without a minimum amount of exercise. You must decide how much exercise you are willing to do and record it.

Exercise is the most important way to increase your metabolism, but a special insulin sensitivity to sugar can possibly mimic a slow metabolism. If you checked "NO" to question (1) in the beginning of chapter 1, this is a possibility. Pay special attention to item 9 in the checklist.

A lack of B vitamins can sometimes slow down your metabolism a little. If you had previously decided not to take vitamins, I hope you will change your mind now. However, taking amounts above what is recommended will not increase your metabolism any further.

Item 8

Some people thrive on stress; others find that it causes distress. You must be the judge in determining how much of your life is affected by stress that becomes distress. Stress robs your body of vitamins, however, if you are already taking vitamins, additional amounts will not do anything about your stress situation.

But there are a number of actions you can take. Identifying

the stressors in your life and evaluating possible countermeasures is a first step in learning how to deal with stress. Instead of getting yourself all upset over something that may only be a molehill, you must learn how to deal with reality. Who suffers when you allow yourself to be put under distress? Only you! If this is difficult for you to overcome, read *Stress Without Distress* by Hans Selye or enroll in a stress-management seminar.

Another method to reduce stress is good planning of your daily activities. Realize what you can handle in the time you have available. This sort of planning should be aimed at ensuring that you get enough rest, especially when you have important activities planned.

Remember, being able to handle the stress in your life means reducing stress-induced hunger mechanisms.

Some people call it stress, others call it a challenge. No matter what you call it, if it changes into distress, you have a negative force in your life. According to several studies by Hans Selye, exercise relieves distress and anxiety. This only becomes important if you have not yet decided to exercise. If you are just starting with a daily exercise program, make sure you have scheduled it so as not to make it a stress factor in your life. Don't force exercise into your daily schedule if you are already exhausted or if you have a very long, hard schedule ahead of you. Plan your exercise so that you have time to do it, and later, allow some time for some extra rest.

Item 9

This point becomes extremely important if you scored more than 35 points on the Harper Health Indicator Test (chapter 9) or if you decided earlier that you have a slow metabolism. We are dealing here with two separate possibilities. You may have some general low blood-sugar problems, or you may have a special insulin sensitivity. Let's talk about the special insulin sensitivity first.

As we pointed out in chapter 9, a special insulin sensitivity can almost totally block your body from burning fat. You can reduce calories more and more, yet if you don't lose any weight, you may assume that you have a very slow metabolism.

To check if this is your problem, go to question (1) on the first page of chapter 1. If your answer was "NO" to this question, there is only one action to help solve this mystery: You must eliminate *all* sugar from your diet; you must check for any hidden sugar in your foods; you cannot have any sweet fruits, not even dried fruits such as raisins. You must also increase lean protein in every meal. Then, if your problem is insulin sensitivity, you will immediately start shedding weight. This is often the case with people who suffer from binging or bulimia.

General low blood-sugar problems are much more common and less serious. If you scored more than 35 points on the Harper Health Indicator Test, you should have your blood-sugar level checked by a prevention-oriented doctor for a possible problem.

In order of decreasing priorities, there are four major actions you should take:

1. Reduce sugar and refined carbohydrates in your diet as much as you can.

2. Exercise to increase lean muscle mass. Lean muscle mass burns calories and serves as a buffer against blood-sugar imbalances because it stores glucose in the form of glycogen.

3. Make sure that you eat some lean protein in every meal; this also helps to achieve blood-sugar homeostasis. Use protein drinks between meals.

4. Take a GTF supplement. GTF contains the mineral chromium and helps to normalize blood sugar regulating mechanisms.

Check if any one of the actions 1 through 4 have been recommended earlier. If yes, place a star next to them to indicate a priority.

Now take a quick look at the factors that could make your weight loss a failure:

- The high calorie drinker must pay attention to counting calories. Follow the rules in chapter 12. This is really a simple problem that can be solved through action. (Item 3a becomes very important.)

- If food allergies are indicated, have your allergies checked or at least go on the four-day rotation diet. Don't ignore the findings.
- An unstable appetite represents a more serious situation. If you suffer from binging or bulimia, read chapter 13 repeatedly and rearrange your priorities as outlined. Consider getting professional help from a nutrition-oriented psychologist or psychiatrist and/or use *The Weight and Appetite-Control Workbook* we recommended in chapter 13.

To fill in the blanks

At the end of your anti-aging weight-loss checklist, there are a number of empty spaces. You can fill in any action that you may find very helpful in achieving your weight goal.

We also have a number of helpful suggestions.

Protein drink. Have half a glass of a protein drink in between meals. This is very important for people with blood-sugar problems or an unstable appetite. If you combine high-fiber foods with a protein drink, this can take the place of a whole meal.

Evening plans. If, like most people, you work a regular job, the time you have available for yourself may be very limited, and if you make plans for the evening, there probably is no time to exercise. However, try to set aside certain evenings devoted just to an exercise program. After exercising, plan time to relax by watching TV, reading a good book, and then going to bed early. You'll feel fantastic the next day.

When you go out for dinner, be sure to follow our nutrition rules and sneak in a little activity afterward by taking a friend for a walk.

Sexual activity. "People who exercise have better sex lives." In general this is true, but it is definitely wrong to assume that strong exercise immediately before sex improves your performance or the pleasure. During the sex act, men and women use a large number of muscles in their bodies. If these muscles are tired and stressed from doing exercise, it will definitely affect your sex life. A good way to improve your sex life with exercise is to go to the gym on a day when you have time and can relax. Then, rest well. You will find that sex the next day is much more satisfying.

Prepared for the urge to snack? Let's face it, we are creatures of habit. For many, a walk into the kitchen automatically means opening the refrigerator door. Stick a sign on the refrigerator door: "*No!* There is no reason for you to open this door!" or "Poor calorie counters acquire the figures to prove it," or make a list of things to do as a diversion. The trick is to find a way to break the habit.

But when it becomes too difficult to resist and we open the door anyway, there must be something safe in there to chew on. Almost all greens and vegetables are appropriate—have some sliced carrot or celery sticks ready; cucumber slices or a salad will also do. There are lots of low-calorie foods that are good for you. Take a stroll through your supermarket and check out the vegetable section. A glass of a prepared protein drink will also help satisfy the need for something. Sip it slowly and make it last, this will prevent low blood sugar levels—as long as you don't drink a whole quart.

Alternatives to eating. You should actually sit down and make a list of things to do: Call a friend, take the dog for a walk, take a walk with a friend, go visit somebody and make sure to tell them not to offer you high-calorie foods, go to a show, clean a closet, read a book, review a chapter in this book, write a letter, organize something, have a facial or your nails done, work on a hobby, take a bubble bath, go out dancing (a great way to burn calories).

Be prepared to have an alternative if the urge to eat hits you.

Time to rest. As you plan your day, make sure that you have sufficient time to rest, especially at night. This is very important for the A-type personality who always pushes for better performance. Plans for the evening? Relax a little! Take a shower, watch some TV, allow yourself a 30-minute nap; these things work wonders and give you a quick recharge.

CONCLUSION

Every day, check each item in the checklist. Be honest. Reevaluate your priorities if your weight loss is not as desired. Look at the day ahead and plan it well.

Don't be too eager to make changes. There will be days when even though you've worked hard on your weight-loss program, the scale will suggest that you haven't lost any weight. This is quite normal. A little water retention, caused by an allergy, a cold, or a delayed bowel movement, can cause a little weight that will disappear the next day. This is quite normal. Just keep plugging along. Don't give up. Your overall shape and your body measurements are often better indicators of your success than just the bathroom scale.

Think about the many anti-aging factors that have entered your life with our program. They are already delaying your aging process; in some instances they can even reverse the signs of aging. Think about your more positive and elevated mood; it's a free bonus that comes with many of the anti-aging measures.

Trust me and follow this program for at least six weeks. You have nothing to lose but weight.

AND NOW KEEP DOING IT!

DON'T GIVE UP!

THE EFFORT IS WORTH IT!

18

HOME COOKING, EATING OUT, PRE-
PACKAGED MEALS: How to make food preparation easy for you.

> Not telling your patients exactly how to
> prepare and choose foods can be the biggest
> stumbling block in a person's weight-loss
> program.
>
> Susan Smith Jones, Ph.D.
> Author of *The Main Ingredient*

At this point in your anti-aging weight-loss program you
should know:

1. What your average daily caloric intake should be in
order to guarantee the desired weight loss.

2. At what frequency and time to consume the foods; not to
skip meals and not to eat large quantities late at night.

3. Which foods to eat and which ones to avoid.

Our next step now is to make it easy for you to prepare or
choose your meals.

Where do you consume your meals? At home? Or do you eat
out most of the time? If you eat at home, do you actually
prepare your meals carefully, or do you just prepare quick
meals such as sandwiches or other snacks? Perhaps you don't
like to cook at all, but you like to use prepackaged meals.

No matter where and how you eat, we have a set of sugges-

217

tions for you. By eating good food, you'll be able to make the food calories count.

IF YOU DON'T COOK BUT EAT OUT

In chapter 3 we gave you a set of food tables (Tables 3.1–3.3). Please take another look at them now.

You'll notice that if you consume the amounts of foods we recommend, the total daily caloric intake is only about 800 calories. *Your* daily caloric allowance is probably several hundred calories higher, and therefore, you can add a few extra calories in terms of using some butter, having a drink, or eating some of the "forbidden foods" from Table 3.1. As we previously pointed out, you don't have to be perfect, just be reasonable.

Whether you prepare some quick foods at home or you eat out most of the time, use these food tables as your guidelines in choosing the right foods. At the end of this chapter, we have included "Hints for eating out." As you develop a sense for "good food," you can add additional references to your list. Pass it along to a friend.

The emphasis is on

- Having some lean protein with every meal
- Eating "low-fat foods" (but don't avoid all fats)
- Avoiding sugar and refined carbohydrates as much as possible, depending on the recommendations that come out of Figure 10.1
- Consuming lots of low-calorie greens

Don't forget, copy Tables 3.1 through 3.3 and take them along for reference.

In combination with your exercise program, you now adjust your food intake so that the desired (reasonable!) weight loss is achieved.

Even if you don't cook, learning to eat right is very important for everyone, so take a look at the meal recommendations that are given at the end of this chapter. Make sure that you understand why the specific foods are combined to make up the complete meals.

IF YOU LIKE PREPACKAGED MEALS

Quite frankly, if you look in the frozen food section of a supermarket and compare the actual food content to what you should be eating, you'll find that a tremendous amount of junk can be found there, and that often the price you pay for these low-quality foods is outrageous.

For years nutrition-oriented health professionals have been telling the food industry that nutritious meals can be low in calories and inexpensive. They rarely listened.

With all the emphasis on low-calorie meals, some big food producers now provide prepackaged wholesome foods that contain vegetables, whole grains, low-fat proteins and low-sugar foods. The results are meal combinations that range from 250 calories to 300 calories per meal. These meals are not exactly what one would define as "supernutritious," but they are reasonable and can be very helpful for people who have to count calories.

These foods are found in the frozen-food section of your health-food store or supermarket. Since natural, unprocessed foods are used, food additives can be kept to a minimum. Read the label; does it sound like the inventory of a chemical laboratory? If yes, then just choose another brand.

One very successful line of frozen low-calorie foods is made by Stouffer's® and is sold under the general name LEAN CUISINE®. This is an excellent product.

If you need more combinations, use the Weight Watchers® prepacked meals. They have also been redesigned and fit into our program.

There are other companies that make similar low-calorie meals. Make certain that you compare the caloric content; even if it says "low-cal" on the label, this doesn't always mean that the meal is truly low in calories.

If you use these prepackaged meals, combine them with other quality foods from Tables 3.1 and 3.2 to arrive at your required daily caloric intake.

At the end of this chapter, we designed a number of daily meal suggestions that are combined with the Stouffer's "Lean

Cuisine" dinner selections. We believe that these entrees are
the only acceptable choices for now.

(*Not for the cook in the family only!* Even if you don't like to
cook, check these meals to understand our nutritional principles.)

Again, in preparing your meals, use Tables 3.1 and 3.2 as
guidelines. Combine the foods to make up complete meals.
Use spices and herbs for flavoring and good taste; the caloric
contents of these flavoring agents are so low that they are
negligible. When preparing a full meal, you want to take into
account

1. Total number of calories
2. Volume of the foods (to fill the stomach)
3. Fat content (overall should be low)
4. Possible refined-carbohydrate (sugar) content
5. Protein (very important—some should be included in
every meal)

From your check items in the table of weight-loss priorities,
you know which factors you have to emphasize. To make it
easier for you, we have included meal suggestions that are
designed for a person whose ideal weight is an average 120
pounds to 160 pounds. Depending on which side of the scale
your weight falls on, you should either consume a little bit less
(if your ideal weight is 120 lb or less), or you can be a little bit
more generous (if your ideal weight is 150 lb or more). Next to
the meal, we list the total calories for the entire meal. We also
list the calories for the single food items.

"Fat" after a food item means that this is the food that you
are to watch (or even reduce further) if you are concerned
about the total fat content in your food and/or if you want to
reduce your overall caloric intake.

"Volume" means that this food item is bulky and fills your
stomach with only a few calories. Increase these foods for
vitamins, minerals, and to give you a "full" feeling. Watch

that these foods are not prepared with other high-calorie foods such as butter.

"Sugar" means that these foods are the ones that possibly contain undesired amounts of refined carbohydrates or sugar. Watch that there is no hidden sugar in the foods you consume. A small amount is relatively unimportant, but as we have seen in chapter 9, it can be a major obstacle in the weight-loss program of some people. Reduce these foods if you checked item 9 in the table of weight-loss priorities.

"Protein" indicates an important food. Protein should be lean and a certain amount should be part of every meal. Protein is important for maintaining normal brain chemistry, to prevent muscle loss, and to keep blood-sugar levels within the normal range.

BUT I NEVER EAT BREAKFAST

For the people who don't like to eat breakfast, you can make yourself a breakfast drink—it's easy and it's fast. Even if you don't like to eat, liquids go down easier and you can develop a variety of flavors that you can enjoy by using your favorite fruit from Table 3.1. If you cannot drink the entire amount, drink half and drink the remainder as a midmorning snack. The caloric content will range from 260 calories to 320 calories per large glass.

All breakfast combinations contain one or more protein foods, one or more servings of roughage foods, and some fluids. There is some fat in eggs, low-fat milk, butter (limit intake) or the cream (use very little). The roughage foods (cereals, fruits, and vegetables) mainly supply carbohydrates.

We would rather you eat the whole fruit instead of drinking its juice because the fruit will increase the amount of roughage, and it will reduce the rate at which the sugar content ends up in the blood as blood sugar.

Since sugar causes so many problems, we have eliminated it from the meals. Even though artificial sweeteners are not yet proven safe, we'd rather have you use them instead of pure sugar. A compromise would be to use a very small amount of honey; one tablespoon has 65 calories. Waffles and pancakes are also not recommended because, again, they are usually consumed with lots of sugary syrup.

If you still always feel hungry, increase your breakfast a little. Try to determine which of the following gives you a "full" feeling: either an increase in the volume of roughage foods or just a small increase in the amount of fat foods.

If you object to the fruit in your diet, increase the other roughage foods a little or buy yourself some roughage tablets such as bran or apple pectin tablets.

WHEN TO TAKE YOUR SUPPLEMENTS

Breakfast is the best time to take all of your supplements except vitamin E and selenium. These two should be taken at night. This has nothing to do with sex, but vitamin E and selenium might help you to rest up in a little less time than is usually required because they may lower your metabolism. Don't take B vitamins at night because they are energy vitamins and might keep you awake.

LUNCH GUIDELINES

To lose weight, there is one major rule you should follow: Stay away from fast-food places (see "Hints for Eating Out" at the end of this chapter). As we have seen in the nutrition chapter, the foods served at these places are extremely high in calories, fats, and sugar.

Many people who work in the health field often have a very small lunch. We also eat dinner at an early hour, around 6 P.M., and therefore, a small lunch is sufficient. This is also the time to take the B and C vitamins if you are on program 2 (chapter 6).

Some of my own lunch examples:

1. 1 thick slice of 9-grain bread with natural peanut butter, 1 apple, 1 glass of mineral water
2. 1 low-fat yogurt with some fresh fruit, 1 slice of whole-grain bread, 1 pear, possibly 1 glass of fruit juice (diluted with mineral water)
3. 1 avocado, 1 small can of sardines in water, 1 thick slice of whole-grain bread, 1 glass of diluted fruit juice.

These small lunches have about 200 calories to 300 calories. There is no sugar in these foods, the protein is of a high quality, and roughage is abundant. Also, the overall fat content is low.

In general, you should combine lots of vegetables, from salads to celery sticks or carrot sticks or any raw vegetable from Table 3.1, with a protein food (low in fat), some whole-grain bread, and low-calorie liquids. The liquids, if possible, should be made with a high-quality drinking water. Try to cut down on your total caffeine consumption, or drink decaffeinated coffee or tea. Include herbal teas and other healthy noncaloric drinks.

BREAKFASTS

These are sample food combinations. You can substitute similar foods from one suggested menu to another.

#1   *Total calories—230*

    1 boiled egg, or fried with very little or no fat (80, protein)

    1 slice whole-grain bread (60, sugar, volume); some of these breads are made with added sugar, or are just high in fiber (read the label)

    ½ grapefruit (45, volume)

    Coffee w/very small amount of cream (20), without cream (0), no sugar

    ½ pat butter (25, fat)

#2 *Total calories—280*
   ¾ C low-fat milk (90)
   2/3 C cornflakes, no sugar added by you (110, sugar)
   1 apple or 1 pear, fresh (80, volume)
   Coffee, black (0)

#3 *Total calories—245*
   1 slice protein bread (35, volume)
   2 scrambled eggs (180, protein)
   Tomato slices (30, volume)
   Coffee, black (0)

#4 *Total calories—275*
   1 C shredded wheat (80, volume)
   1 wedge watermelon (100, sugar)
   ½ C low-fat milk (60, protein, fat)
   2 T low-fat cottage cheese (35, protein)
   Coffee, black (0)

#5 *Total calories—340*
   2 poached eggs (160, protein)
   1 slice whole-grain bread (60, volume)
   1 T peanut butter (70, protein) (avoid common brands that have hidden sugar, be sure label says peanuts only)
   ½ C orange juice (50, sugar)

Note: Coffee (or tea) is not a requirement for any breakfast. You may have herbal tea, mineral water, or water with a noncaloric healthy fizz tablet added.

LUNCHES

#1 *Total calories—330*
   Tuna salad sandwich
     6 oz tuna salad, water packed (150 protein)
     2 slices whole-grain bread (120, volume)
     Small amount mayonnaise (30, fat)
     Lettuce, tomato (30, volume)
   Coffee or a diet drink

#2   *Total calories—350*
Small chef's salad
   1 egg, hard boiled (80, protein)
   1 oz chicken (40, protein)
   1 oz boiled ham (70, protein, fat)
   2 C mixed greens (30, volume)
   1 T dressing (70, fat, sugar)
1 slice whole-grain bread (60, volume)
Coffee or a diet drink (0)

#3   *Total calories—310*
Other similar small salad
   Greens, meat, dressing (similar to #2 without chicken)
Bread
Coffee or a diet drink

#4   *Total calories—370*
Vegetable plate, cooked w/cheese
   Vegetables (150, volume)
   2 oz cheese sauce (100, protein, fat)
1 pat butter (50, fat)
1 slice protein bread (35, volume)
7 oz regular carbonated beverage, 50% club soda (35, sugar)

#5   *Total calories—340*
Chicken soup (or similar soup) (140, protein, fat)
2 oz lean beef patty (150, protein, fat)
1 slice whole-grain bread, no sugar added (60, volume)
Coffee or a diet drink (0)

Note: Coffee (or tea) or a diet drink is not a requirement for any lunch. You may have herbal tea or mineral water.

DINNERS

These are sample food combinations for people who enjoy preparing their own meals. You can exchange similar foods from one suggestion to another.

#1 *Total calories—300*
4 oz chicken, well-done, broiled (110, protein)
1 C broccoli, steamed; 1 t butter, some garlic powder (70, volume, fat)
½ C mushrooms, steamed (30, volume)
¼ oz parmesan cheese sprinkled over vegetables (30, protein)
Fruit juice diluted with club soda (30, sugar)
½ whole-wheat muffin (30, volume)

#2 *Total calories—360*
4 oz fish, broiled or baked (90, protein)
6 spears asparagus, 1 t butter (50, volume, fat)
1 small mixed salad, w/small amount dressing (60, volume)
1 slice whole-wheat bread (60, volume)
1 pat butter (50, fat)
1 glass wine spritzer (50, sugar)

#3 *Total calories—380*
3 oz steak, well-done (260, protein)
1 C carrots, steamed (35, volume)
Mixed salad, low-calorie dressing (50, volume)
1 slice protein bread (35, volume)
Coffee or diet drink

Note: Coffee (or tea) or a diet drink is not a requirement for any dinner. You may have herbal tea. mineral water, or plain water with a noncaloric fizz tablet added.

SAMPLE MENU #1

Women: 1200 calories   Men: 1600 calories

Breakfast

2/3 C oat bran or dry cereal	½ C orange juice
½ C 2% milk	2/3 C oat bran or dry cereal
1 soft-boiled egg	½ C 2% milk

1 small banana or peach	1 soft-boiled egg
Coffee or tea	1 medium banana or peach
	1 slice whole-grain toast
	2 t butter
	Coffee or tea

Lunch

Ham & cheese sandwich	Ham & cheese sandwich
1 oz Swiss cheese	2 oz Swiss cheese
1½ oz boiled ham	2 oz boiled ham
Lettuce and mustard	Lettuce and mustard
2 slices whole-grain bread	2 slices whole brain bread
Carrot and celery sticks	Carrot and celery sticks
1 small orange	1 medium orange
Broth or mineral water	Broth or mineral water

*Dinner**

Stouffer's *Lean Cuisine*	Stouffer's *Lean Cuisine*
Filet of Fish Divan with	*Filet of Fish Divan with*
Broccoli®	*Broccoli*®

Add the following if you wish:

1 slice whole-grain bread	1 slice whole-grain bread
½ C blueberries	¾ C blueberries
Herbal tea	Herbal tea

Note: Whenever possible, select foods from a health-food store. Read all labels to avoid sugar, salt, flour (used for thickeners), artificial color, and preservatives.

SAMPLE MENU #2

Women: 1200 calories	Men: 1600 calories

Breakfast

1 small orange or	1 small orange or
½ grapefruit	½ grapefruit

*These four dinner suggestions are for those who don't wish to prepare their own meals.

1 scrambled egg	2 scrambled eggs
1 slice whole-grain toast or	1 slice whole-grain toast or
1 slice raisin toast	1 slice raisin toast
1 pat butter	1 pat butter
Coffee or tea	Coffee or tea

Lunch

1 C beef broth	1 C beef noodle soup
Roast beef or turkey	Roast beef or turkey
sandwich	sandwich
2 oz lean meat	3 oz lean meat
2 slices whole-grain bread	2 slices whole-grain bread
1 T mayonnaise	1 T mayonnaise
1 small tomato	1 small tomato
1 small pear	1 medium pear
1 C 2% milk	1 C 2% milk
4 oz vegetable juice	4 oz vegetable juice

Dinner

Stouffer's *Lean Cuisine*   Stouffer's *Lean Cuisine*
Chicken & Vegetables with   *Chicken & Vegetables with*
Vermicelli®   *Vermicelli*®

  Add the following for more bulk and few calories:

Tossed green salad	Tossed green salad
1 C mixed greens	1 C mixed greens
Sliced cucumber	Sliced cucumber
1 T low-cal dressing	1 T low-cal dressing
(25 cal)	(25 cal)
1 C melon balls	1 C melon balls
Herbal tea	Herbal tea

Note: Whenever possible, select foods as fresh as possible. Read all labels to avoid sugar, salt, flour (used for thickener), artificial colors, and preservatives.

SAMPLE MENU #3

Women: 1200 calories   Men: 1600 calories

Breakfast

½ C orange juice	½ C orange juice
2/3 C oatmeal or dry cereal	2/3 C oatmeal or dry cereal
1 C 2% milk	1 C 2% milk
1 T raisins	1 T raisins
1 soft-boiled egg	1 soft-boiled egg
Coffee or tea	1 slice whole-grain toast
	1 t butter
	Coffee or tea

Lunch

Chef's salad	Chef's salad
2 C tossed greens	2 C tossed greens
chilled raw vegetables	chilled raw vegetables
1 small tomato	1 small tomato
3 oz total: chicken, turkey, cheese	5 oz total: chicken, turkey, cheese
2 T low-cal dressing (50 cal)	2 T regular dressing
1 small whole-grain dinner roll	1 small whole-grain dinner roll
1 small orange or tangerine	1 t butter
1 C 2% milk	1 medium orange or tangerine
Mineral water w/lime wedge	1 C 2% milk
	Mineral water w/lime wedge

Dinner

Stouffer's *Lean Cuisine Zucchini Lasagna*®	Stouffer's *Lean Cuisine Zucchini Lasagna*®

Add the following for more bulk and few calories:

Chilled raw vegetables carrots, broccoli, celery, cauliflower, etc.	Chilled raw vegetables carrots, broccoli, celery, cauliflower, etc.
¼ C low-fat cottage cheese dip	¼ C low-fat cottage cheese dip
½ C strawberries	¾ C strawberries
Herbal tea	Herbal tea

Low-fat cottage cheese dip
¼ C low-fat cottage cheese
2 drops Worcestershire
   sauce
⅛ t parsley
1 drop tabasco sauce
Garlic powder, pepper,
   oregano, basil to taste

Mix all ingredients thoroughly

Note: Whenever possible, select foods from a health-food
   store. Read all labels to avoid sugar, salt, flour (used for
   thickener), artificial colors, and preservatives.

SAMPLE MENU #4

Women: 1200 calories   Men: 1600 calories

Breakfast

Women	Men
¼ small cantaloupe or ½ C apple juice	¼ small cantaloupe or ½ C apple juice
1 whole-wheat toasted bagel or 1 whole-wheat English muffin	1 whole-wheat toasted bagel or 1 whole-wheat English muffin
3 T peanut butter	4 T peanut butter
Coffee or tea	1 t butter
	Coffee or tea

Lunch

Women	Men
1 C beef-vegetable soup	1 C beef-vegetable soup
Fruit salad	Fruit salad
1 C mixed fruit	1 C mixed fruit
¾ C low-fat cottage cheese	1 C low-fat cottage cheese
Crisp greens	Crisp greens
1 T low-cal dressing	1 T regular dressing
6 whole-wheat crackers	6 whole-wheat crackers
4 oz tomato juice	1 C 2% milk
	4 oz tomato juice

Dinner

Stouffer's *Lean Cuisine*   Stouffer's *Lean Cuisine*
  Oriental Beef in Sauce &   *Oriental Beef in Sauce &*
  Vegetables with Rice®   *Vegetables with Rice®*

Add the following for more bulk and few calories:

½ C steamed or raw carrots   ½ C steamed or raw carrots
12 grapes   1 small whole wheat dinner
Herbal tea   roll
                         1 t butter
                         12 grapes
                         Herbal tea

Note: Whenever possible, select foods from a health-food store. Read all labels to avoid sugar, salt, flour (used for thickeners), artificial colors, and preservatives.

HINTS FOR EATING OUT

You might want to make a photocopy of this page and keep it with you to help you select the *right* foods. When you have a choice, avoid fast-food chains and stick to health-oriented restaurants. If it is not possible, here is what you should do:

- At breakfast, order oatmeal instead of high-calorie pancakes or waffles.
- At the cocktail hour, ask for mineral water with lime. This has become socially acceptable.
- Select roasted or broiled meat, chicken, or fish; never fried or breaded.
- Request whole-wheat bread or rolls.
- Salads are almost always available. Request dressing on the side so that you can control the quantity (be conservative).
- If the choices are really high calorie, eggs are a good high-protein, low-calorie food for any meal; poached is lowest in calories.
- Avoid foods with sauces.
- Substitute tomatoes or cottage cheese for potatoes or ask

for plain baked potatoes (without any butter or sour cream).

- Get in the habit of refusing desserts. (Remember how stuffed you felt?) Instead, have fresh fruit.
- Ask for herbal tea. Many restaurants now carry a choice of teas.

It's really easy once you develop a habit. Your friends will envy your willpower and your health.

19

CONGRATULATIONS

You have worked your way up to this point, and now you know what you must do to lose those pounds, to get into shape, and to rejuvenate yourself. It will take some effort but just dig in and be patient. The rewards will be tremendous; you will really fall in love with our approach when you recognize that the unwanted pounds will stay off.

As you move along and follow your personal weight-loss program, make sure you use the weight-loss checklist every day. When you weigh yourself every morning, compare your weight loss to your weight-loss actions during the last few days; you will soon notice a relationship. Keep a close eye on them. Because of your biochemical individuality, you might notice that some weight-loss factors work especially well for you. At this point, some people have a tendency to follow only these weight-loss factors. Although this might work for some

people, it will definitely spell weight-loss failure for others.
You can emphasize and stress weight-loss factors that work
well for you, but make sure never to completely drop any one
of your required weight-loss actions.

THIS IS A GOOD TIME TO REVIEW

Never assume that you know everything after going
through this book just once. Remember, we are also building a
basis for the best possible long-term health. From time to
time review the first nine chapters. Often, when you read
something for the second time, it will suddenly become clear,
and you will see why certain recommendations are truly
necessary. Read through a previous chapter even if you think
that you already understand it. At the Health Integration
Center in Torrance, California, where we conduct weight-loss
and eating-disorder counseling, we always give reading
assignments of previously covered material. Then we review
the subjects with the patients to make sure that everything is
totally understood. It might sound boring, but it certainly
gives excellent results. Once you understand the principles
behind our advice, you will be able to utilize them to make
correct decisions in any given situation.

YOU MUST UNDERSTAND THAT THERE IS NO EASIER WAY

Some people, when they recognize that it requires some
effort, are tempted to give up and change to the latest adver-
tised diet gimmick. No matter what the promoters promise
you, don't give in!
At the time of the writing of this book, a number of companies were working on some natural appetite suppressants;
they were supposed to contain no drugs, just herbs or other
natural nutrients. Should one of these new products become
available in the meantime, you can include it in your program
to help you cut down on your total food intake, but never quit
our weight-loss program in favor of any new miracle pill.

One thing is for sure: People who give up for any reason remain fat, and people who endure and work at their program get results. We see this every day, not only in respect of weight loss, but also in relation to general health and chronic diseases. People who don't take preventive action and who rely on the outdated drug approach usually die at an average age, feeling and looking old at a far too early stage in their lives. People who take charge of their own health are the ones with "success" written all over their faces.

One of the pioneers of holistic health, Gaylord Hauser, died recently at age 89. Just a few years ago I had met him, and I recalled somebody saying that he was 65 at that time. I was very impressed and thought to myself: "I hope that I'll look as good at age 65." Later, when I found out that he was really 85 years old at the time that I met him, I was truly amazed. Can you imagine how long he would have lived, and how young he could have looked, had he known all the anti-aging possibilities at an earlier stage in his life?

HOLISTIC MEDICINE GETS SOME ORTHODOX DOCTORS NERVOUS

The principles of holistic health and medicine are still quite new to many people, even to some health professionals. It was long accepted that certain risk factors such as smoking, lack of exercise, and excessive food intake could bring on diseases such as diabetes, cancer, and heart ailments. Then, a few years ago, medical publications started to demonstrate that even simple nutritional factors could delay or prevent chronic diseases. Most recently, it was demonstrated that these and other health factors also worked in the treatment of the chronic diseases we mentioned above.

Even this frightens some old-fashioned doctors who can't accept progress; they are afraid that medicine is being taken out of their hands. Many orthodox doctors who practice crisis medicine still adhere to the school of thought—which in many instances has already been proved wrong—that for every disease there must be a drug to cure it. Driven by their fears,

and often financially supported by special interests, you can
see questionable scientists making all kinds of distorted or
untrue statements about holistic health.

Then there are the health professionals who simply warn
you that all these holistic health methods have not yet been
researched enough, and they express an opinion even though
it is obvious that they are not up-to-date about what is being
published in the medical literature.

And then there are the professors of medicine who have
learned a few tricks about show business and ridicule everything, from hair analysis to vitamin supplements. Sometimes
they make totally incorrect statements that are not recognized as such by the audience. For example, when asked
about hair analysis, they may reply: "There is no single publication in the medical literature that proves that it helps in
determining people's vitamin needs. Only charlatans would
tell you that." A person listening to such comments might
think that hair analysis is a charlatan practice. As a matter of
fact, nobody in the holistic health field will ever tell you that
hair analysis is used to determine your vitamin needs. The
analysis tells you only about the mineral status in your body,
which mineral supplements you need, and which toxic minerals might affect your health. So, although these people
haven't told a lie, they sure have confused the audience. Why
do they do that? Even people like the Nobel Prize winner
Linus Pauling have asked this question without getting an
answer.

At other times, you might hear a university professor warn
you that taking vitamin C can be dangerous because he found
evidence in his research that it destroys vitamin B_{12} and that
you might risk anemia. Sounds pretty bad for vitamin C,
doesn't it? Relax! His suggestions have already been proved
wrong in medical publications; there is even a famous
research group from a pharmaceutical company that repeated the experiments and suggested that the professor
goofed in his research and used the wrong laboratory techniques. Naturally, the good professor doesn't tell you about
these findings and instead of taking more care with his

future research, he recently published another such research paper. His "research" was repeated by a famous FDA-approved laboratory, and we are again being told that his research data are incorrect. By knowing your facts, you will never be impressed by questionable scientists.

HAVE WE REACHED OUR GOAL?

Please understand that this book was not supposed to be an encyclopedia of all weight-loss programs or all anti-aging measures that were ever proposed. These topics have been discussed elsewhere.

Our goal was to give you a weight-loss program that works, that doesn't include unnecessary procedures, that avoids all the causes of premature aging often associated with weight-loss diets, and that includes the best anti-aging measures.

I hope you will agree that we have reached this goal.

KEEP US INFORMED

In order for future weight-loss programs to be even more successful, let us know how you fared with The Anti-Aging Weight-Loss Program. Appendix A is a questionnaire that we would like you to complete. Take a minute to fill in the basic information right now. Then, after six weeks on our program, complete it and return it to us. It will help us in many ways. In appreciation of your efforts, we will inform you if something new and important should be discovered that might change our weight-loss approach.

Take charge of your health.

Take charge of your life.

Appendix A

Return to: Health Integration Center
            3250 Lomita Blvd. Suite 208
            Torrance, CA 90505
            Attn. Dr. Kugler

Mr.
Mrs. _____   Age: _____
Ms.

Address: _____   Sex: _____

City: _____   Height: _____

State: _____ Zip: _____   Weight
                                     at start: _____

                                     Weight after
                                     6 weeks: _____

239

Which ones of the weight-loss
factors (chap. nos.) were especially
helpful to you?   _____

Which weight-loss factors (chap.
nos.) were least important to you?   _____

How many weight-loss diets   How many diet books
have you tried in the   have you read in the
past _____ years? _____   past _____ years? _____

Do you have an eating disorder? Bulimia ____ Binging ____

Did you involve your doctor? ____

A psychologist/psychiatrist? _____

Your condition and/or symptoms before you started the
Anti-aging Weight-Loss Program:

What is your opinion about the Anti-Aging Weight-Loss Program?

Appendix B

Where you can get your body fat measured without charge. In chapter 2 we mentioned an agreement with a number of health clubs. Call for an appointment for a first visit, tell them that you want your body fat measured, and take this book along and show it to them. We are not responsible if any of the clubs does not have the tables to measure body fat according to Dr. Katch. The participating clubs are:

California: Holiday Spa Health Clubs
Colorado: Holiday Health and Fitness Centers
Connecticut: American Health and Fitness Centers
Florida (north): Bally North Florida
Georgia: Holiday Health and Fitness Centers

Illinois: Chicago Health Clubs; Chicago Fair Lady; North Shore Club

Maryland: U.S. Health and Recreation; Holiday Health Spas

Michigan: Vic Tanny International

Missouri: Vic Tanny International

Ohio: Vic Tanny International; Scandinavian Holiday Health Spas

New Jersey: Jack LaLane; European Health Spa

New York: Jack LaLanne of New York; (Long Island) Holiday Spa Health Clubs; (New York City) The Vertical Club; American Health and Fitness Centers

Pennsylvania: American Health and Fitness Centers; Holiday Health Spas

Rhode Island: American Health and Fitness Centers

South Carolina: Holiday Health and Fitness Centers

Texas: President's First Lady; Dallas Health Clubs; President's Health Clubs

Virginia: Holiday Health and Fitness Centers

Wisconsin: Vic Tanny International; Vic Tanny Health Clubs

Also Richard Simmons Anatomy Asylums. These clubs use the RJL method discussed in chapter 2, and they might charge you a few dollars for measuring body fat. Call and ask them about it before you go there.

Appendix C

For the beginner: To make your exercise start easy and without risk.

The advisory board of the Chicago Health Clubs and the Tennis Corporation of America, which includes leading specialists in the areas of health and physical recreation, has worked out a list of do's and don'ts that summarizes the most basic rules for a good exercise program.

Follow these directions. The right exercise program will help you to improve your energy, endurance, and resistance to diseases, while extending your life expectancy. Exercise is also a key factor in losing weight, maintaining cardiovascular fitness, and preventing the formation of cellulite.

TRAINING TIPS FROM THE ADVISORY BOARD
HEALTH AND TENNIS CORPORATION OF AMERICA*

Preface: Exercise can and should be enjoyable! Exercise
is a natural and safe way to improve health, promote
physical fitness and enhance the enjoyment of life. Exercise can help to improve appearance, help reduce excess
fat and help to improve abilities in recreational activities
and athletic participation.

The following training tips will insure that you get the
most out of your exercise program in a safe and effective
way. These principles are applicable to normal healthy
individuals of both sexes at all ages.

DO's
1. DO make exercise a regular habit. Set aside a
   specific time during the day as you would for eating
   and sleeping.
2. DO warm up! Begin each exercise session with 5 to 15
   minutes of light exercises preparing all muscles,
   tendons, and joints for increasingly more vigorous
   activity.
3. DO "cool down" activity during the last 5 minutes of
   each exercise session, using exercises which will help
   to relax all muscles.
4. DO balance your exercise program by including and
   mixing: endurance-type exercises such as walking,
   jogging, running, cycling, and swimming; exercises
   to build up adequate muscle strength; flexibility
   exercises; and exercises to improve motor skills.
5. DO a minimum of three strength and muscle endurance workouts per week. Cardio-Vascular-Respira-
   tory endurance exercises should be performed daily.
6. DO elevate your pulse rate into the range of 130–160
   beats per minute when performing endurance exercise.

*I am grateful to the Chicago Health Clubs and the Tennis Corporation of
America for letting me use this material

7. DO keep a daily record of your attendance and exercise efforts and a weekly record of your weight and of any problems encountered.
8. DO periodically evaluate the progress of your physical fitness exercise program.
9. DO, if over 35 years of age, consult with your physician for a physical examination and, most desirable, for a Functional Capacity Test prior to participating in any physical fitness program.
10. DO combine dietary and exercise routines to help maintain a desirable body weight (without excess fat).
11. DO a strength and muscle endurance exercise program that works every major muscle group. It is not wise to use only selected exercises. This can lead to a muscular strength imbalance.

DON'Ts
1. *DON'T* perform any exercise program against the wishes of your physician.
2. *DON'T* exercise vigorously within one hour after any major meal.
3. *DON'T* exercise if you have a common cold, respiratory ailment, specific or unspecific infection, or any other illness or physical handicap—without medical approval.
4. *DON'T* strain to perform an exercise. Increase the intensity of exercise only when it becomes easy.
5. *DON'T* sit or lie down immediately after exercising. Keep moving (at least 10 minutes) to facilitate recovery from your previous efforts.
6. *DON'T* use rubber suits, rubber belts, whirlpool, steam, and sauna baths as a means of attempting to lose weight. These devices merely dehydrate the body and do not burn up the excess body fat.
7. *DON'T* abuse your body with excesses of food, alcohol, and nicotine.
8. *DON'T* go on a "fad" diet. A calorically balanced diet, which includes the four basic food groups, is the only

sensible and correct approach to diet and nutrition management.

9. *DON'T* try to reduce more than two pounds per week.

10. *DON'T* use passive exercise equipment such as rollers or vibrators. These devices are not effective for eliminating fat or increasing muscle tone and can be dangerous when used as massaging agents.

11. *DON'T* routinely exercise to the extent of physical discomfort and real pain—but enjoy your physical experiences.

REMEMBER

A sedentary person will begin to feel better after a few workouts. However, it will take a longer time to observe physical and physiological improvements.

Soreness, associated with exercises that are newly performed, may be minimized by starting at lower intensity levels. Progressive adjustment of exercise intensity assures comfortable and continued improvement. Training must be *progressive, regular, frequent*, and sufficiently *vigorous.*

Each individual has a different exercise tolerance. Train within your own tolerance.

The cumulative physiological changes induced by exercise are the very best and most effective means for achieving permanent fat reduction and normalization of body weight. Lack of exercise causes premature physiological aging and deterioration of functional capacity. For best results, exercise must be combined with other good health habits.

Appendix D

To obtain more information, brochures, a sample copy of the H. & P. UP-DATE, computer programs and other services, covering and including hair analysis, weight control, bulimia, videocassettes on aging, and so forth, please send a stamped self-addressed envelope to:

Dr. Hans J. Kugler
International Academy of Holistic Health and Medicine
218 Avenue B
Redondo Beach, CA 90277

References and Notes

Introduction

Strehler, "Aging: Transcriptional and Translational Control Mechanisms and Their Alteration."

Black, et al., "Minimal Interventions for Weight Control; A Cost-effective Alternative."

Jeffery, et al., "Correlates of Weight Loss and Its Maintenance Over Two Years of Follow-up Among Middle-aged Men."

Baanders-van Halewijn, et al., "The Cordon Study of Weight Reduction Based on Behavior Modification."

Hudiburgh, "A Multidisciplinary Approach to Weight Control."

Russ, Ciavarella, and Atkinson, "A Comprehensive Outpatient Weight Reduction Program."

Weinsier, et al., "Recommended Therapeutic Guidelines for Professional Weight Control Programs."

Chapter 1

Passwater, *Supernutrition for Healthy Hearts*. Gives a detailed discussion.

Kugler, *Dr. Kugler's Seven Keys to a Longer Life.*
DeLuise, Blackburn, and Flier, "Reduced Activity of the Red-
    cell Sodium Potassium Pump in Human Obesity."
Webb, "Direct Calorimetry and the Energetics of Exercise
    and Weight Reduction."

Chapter 2
Katch, McArdle, and Boylan, *Getting in Shape.*
Body Composition Analyzer, Model BIAC-103, RJL Systems,
    9930 Whittier, Detroit, MI 48224.
Lukaski, "Assessment of Fat-free Mass Using Bioelectrical
    Impedance Measurements of the Human Body."
Picot, Rolland, and Hellegouarch, "Lean Body Mass and Body
    Fat Evaluation by Electrical Impedancemetry."

Chapter 3
Stern, "Useful Animal Models and Techniques in the Study of
    Exercise and Obesity."
Scrimshaw, "An Analysis of Past and Present Recommended
    Dietary Allowances for Protein in Health and Disease."
Horrobin, et al., "The Nutritional Regulation of T Lympho-
    cyte Function."
Bland, "Serum Lipids, Prostaglandins, and Marine Oils."
Passwater, *The Easy No-Flab Diet*; Kramsch, Aspen, and
    Rozler, "Atherosclerosis: Prevention by Agents Not Af-
    fecting Abnormal Levels of Blood Lipids."
Oscai, "Exercise and Weight Reduction in the Obese Rat."
Nutrition Science Laboratories, P.O. Box 400, Essex, VT
    05451.
For more details about the principles outlined in this chapter,
    see any standard biochemistry and/or nutrition textbook.

Chapter 4
Hylander and Rossner, "Effects of Dietary Fiber Intake
    Before Meals on Weight Loss and Hunger in a Weight-
    reducing Club."

Chen and Anderson, "Effects of Plant Fiber in Decreasing Plasma Total Cholesterol and Increasing High-Density Lipoprotein Cholesterol."

Reubin, *The Save Your Life Diet.*

Burkitt, Walker, and Painter, "Effects of Dietary Fiber on Stool and Transit Times, and Its Role in the Causation of Disease."

Atkins, *Dr. Atkin's Nutritional Breakthrough.*

Chapter 5

Gallup Youth Survey, "Third of Teens Skip Breakfast."

Marston, "Effects of Excessive Caloric Intake and Caloric Restriction on Body Weight and Energy Expenditure at Rest and Light Exercise."

Graeber, R., in *The Woman Doctor's Diet for Women* by Edelstein and *The Easy No-Flab Diet* by Passwater.

Lamb, "Muscle Loss from Weight Loss."

Weindruch, Gottesman, and Walford, "Modification of Age-related Immune Decline in Mice Dietarily Restricted from or after Mid-adulthood."

Carlson and Hoelzel, "Apparent Prolongation of the Life Span of Rats by Intermittent Fasting."

Cheney, et al., "Survival and Disease Patterns in C57BL/6J Mice Subjected to Undernutrition."

Kugler, "Food Frequency Intake, Exercise, and Muscle Mass in Bulimics."

Chapter 6

Cheraskin, Ringsdorf, and Brecher, *Psychodietetics.*

Schrauzer, McGinness, and Kuehn, "Effects of Selenium Supplementation on the Genesis of Spontaneous Mammary Tumors in Inbred C3H/St Mice.

Cheraskin, "Influence of Nutrients on Behavior."

Kugler, "Diet and Health Habits as Related to the Onset of Disease."

Cheraskin, Ringsdorf, and Medford, "The Ideal Daily Vitamin A Intake."

Passwater, *Selenium as Food and Medicine.*

Walford, *Maximum Life Span.*

Horvath and Ip, "Synergistic Effect of Vitamin E and Selenium in the Chemoprevention of Mammary Carcinogenesis in Rats."

Wald, et al., "Plasma Retinol, Beta-carotene, and Vitamin E Levels in Relation to the Future Risk of Breast Cancer."

Belizan, "Reduction of Blood Pressure with Calcium Supplements in Young Adults."

Bull, "Low Calcium, Chlorine, and Fat Linked to Heart Disease."

Belko, et al., "Effects of Aerobic Exercise and Weight Loss on Riboflavin Requirements of Moderately Obese, Marginally Deficient Young Women."

Chapter 7

Morris, et al., "Vigorous Exercise in Leisure-time and the Incidence of Coronary Heart Disease."

Anderson, Kiehm, and Ward, "Beneficial effects of a high carbohydrate, High Fiber Diet on Hyperglycemic Diabetic Men."

Greist, "Exercise in the Prevention and Treatment of Depression."

Kugler, "The Importance of Exercise in the Treatment of Bulimia."

Stern, "Useful Animal Models and Techniques in the Study of Exercise and Obesity."

Horton, "Metabolic aspects of Exercise and Weight Reduction."

Cureton, "Wheat Germ Oil, the 'Wonder' Fuel."

Cureton, "Nutritive Aspects of Physical Fitness Work."

Bland, "Octacosanol, Carnitine and Other 'Accessory' Nutrients."

Graeber, et al., "Immunomodulating Properties of Dimethylglycine in Humans."

DMG (dimethyl glycine): manufactured by Da Vinci Laboratories, 20 New England Dr., Essex Junction, VT 05452.

Food Science Laboratories, 20 New England Dr., Essex Junction, VT 05452.

Inosin-Cardiacum: manufactured by A. S. Biologische und Pharmazeutische Produkte GmbH, Freiburg, W. Germany.

Xobaline: manufacutred by Albert-Roussel Pharma GmbH, Wiesbaden, W. Germany.

Ornish, "Good Health Practices, an Effective Means in Preventing Heart Disease."

Columbu, *Redesign Your Body.*

Pascher, "Die Wasserloeslichen Bestandteile der Peripheren Hornschicht (Hautoberflaeche) Wuantitative Analysen, Pyrrolidoncarbonsaeure."

Middleton and Roberts, "Effect of a Skin Cream Containing the Sodium Salts of Pyrrolidone Carboxylic Acid on Dry and Flaky Skin."

Clar and Fourtanier, "L'acide Pyrrolidone Carboxylique (PCA) et la peau."

Chapter 8

Selye, "Stress and Aging."

Selye, *Stress Without Distress.*

Selye, "Stress, Cancer and Behavior."

Rosch, "Stress and Cardiovascular Disease."

Chapter 9

Cheraskin and Ringsdorf, "Homeostasis: The Crux of the Prevention Problem."

Harper, *How You Can Beat the Killer Diseases.*

Sussman, et al., "Plasma Insulin Levels During Reactive Hypoglycemia."

Hofeldt and Lufkin, "Are abnormalities in Insulin Secretion Responsible for Reactive Hypoglycemia?"

Faserberg, et al., "Weight-reducing Diets: Role of Carbohydrates on Sympathetic Nervous Activity and Hypotensive Response."

Ward, *Emotional Aspects of Hypoglycemia in Endocrinology and Diabetes.*

Yaryura and Neziroglu, "Psychosis and Disturbance of Glucose Metabolism."
Smythies, "The Biochemistry of Psychosis."

Chapter 10
Belloc and Breslow, "Relationship of Physical Health Status
and Health Practices."
Colvin and Olson, "A Descriptive Analysis of Men and
Women Who Have Lost Significant Weight and Are
Highly Successful at Maintaining the Loss."
Sheldahl, "Special Ergometric Techniques and Weight Re-
duction."
Ben, "Is Detoxification a Solution to Occupational Health
Hazards?"
Schnare, "Body Burden Reduction of PCBs, PBBs and Chlor-
inated Pesticides in Human Subjects."
Passwater and Cranton, *Trace Elements, Hair Analysis and
Nutrition.*
Holistic and Preventive UP-DATE, newsletter published by
the International Academy of Holistic Health and Medi-
cine, 218 Avenue B, Redondo Beach, CA 90277.

Chapter 11
American Businessman's Research Foundation, report on
alcohol.
Rodale, "Polluted Rats Turn to Drink."

Chapter 12
Coker, "Cytotoxic Testing."
Grant, "Food Allergy and Migraine."
Reinhardt, "Biochemical Pathology Initiated by Free Radi-
cals, Oxidant Chemicals, and Therapeutic Drugs in the
Etiology of Chemical Hypersensitivity Disease."
Mooney, *The Supernutrition Handbook.*
Allergy Research Review, published by Nutri-Cology.

Chapter 13
Kugler, "Are You a Victim of Bulimia?"
Kugler, *The Weight and Appetite Control Workbook.*
Fairburn, "A Cognitive Behavioral Approach to the Treatment of Bulimia."
Pyle, Mitchell, and Eckert, "Bulimia: A Report of 34 Cases."
Mitchell, Pyle, and Elke, "Frequency and Duration of Binge-eating Episodes in Patients with Bulimia."

Chapter 14
Clayman and O'Reilly, "Jejunoileal Bypass: Pass It By."
Rucker, et al., "Searching for the Best Weight-reduction Operation."
Lampman, "Exercise as a Partial Therapy for the Grossly Obese."
Merimee, et al., "Arginine-initiated Release of Human Growth Hormone."

Chapter 16
Carpenter and Hart, "Toward an Integrated Theory of Aging."
Pearl, *The Rate of Living Theory of Aging.*
McKay, C. M., "Chemical Aspects of Aging and the Effect of Diet upon Aging," in *Cowdry's Problems of Ageing,* edited by Lansing.
Hartman, "The Free Radical Theory of Aging."
Fujimoto, "Aging and Cross-linking in Human Aorta."
Wald, Idle, and Boreham, "Low Serum Vitamin A and Subsequent Risk of Cancer."
Walford, "The Immunologic Theory of Aging."
Cheraskin and Ringsdorf, "Homeostasis: The Crux of the Prevention Problem."
Hager, "Implantation von fetalem Thymusgewebe zur Steigerung der Koerpereigenen Abwehr."
Hayflick, "The Cellular Basis for Biological Aging," in *Hand-*

book of the Biology of Aging, edited by Finch and Hayflick.

Packer and Smith, "Extension of the In-vitro Lifespan of Human WI-38 Cells by Vitamin E."

Still, "A Cybernetic Theory of Aging."

Kugler, "The Combination Theory of Aging."

Breslow and Belloc, "Relationship of Physical Health Status and Health Practices."

Walford, *Maximum Life Span.*

Bibliography

Allergy Research Review. Concord, CA: Nutri-Colgy, 2336-C Stanwell Circle, Concord, CA 94520.

American Businessman's Research Foundation. Report on alcohol. Elmhurst, Illinois: 1971.

Anderson, J. W., T. Kiehm, and K. Ward, "Beneficial Effects of a High Carbohydrate, High Fiber Diet on Hyperglycemic Diabetic Men." *The American Journal of Clinical Nutrition* 8 (1976): 895-99.

Atkins, R., *Dr. Atkin's Nutrition Breakthrough.* New York: Random House, 1976.

Baanders-van Halewijm, E. A., Y. W. Choy, J. van Uitert, and F. de Waard. "The Cordon Study of Weight Reduction Based on Behavior Modification."
Int. J. Obes. 2 (1984): 161-70.

Belizan, J. "Reduction of Blood Pressure with Calcium Supplements in Young Adults." *JAMA* 249 (1983): 1161-65.

Belko, A. Z., E. Obarzanek, R. Roach, M. Rotter, G. Urban, S. Weinberg, and D. A. Roes. "Effects of Aerobic Exercise and Weight Loss on Riboflavin Requirements of Moderately Obese, Marginally Deficient Young Women." *Am. J. Clin. Nutr.* 3 (September 1984): 553-61.

Belloc, N. and L. Breslow. "Relationship of Physical Health
    Status and Health Practices." *Preventive Medicine*, No. 1
    (1972): 409–21.
Ben, M., "Is Detoxification a Solution to Occupational Health
    Hazards?" *National Safety News* (May 1984): 1–2.
Black, D. R., W. C. Coe, J. G. Friesen, and A. G. Wurzman.
    "Minimal Interventions for Weight Control: A Cost-
    effective Alternative." *Addict. Behav.* 3 (1984): 279–85.
Bland, J. S. "Octacosanol, Carnitine and Other 'Accessory'
    Nutrients." New Canaan: Keats Publishing, *The Good
    Health Guide* series, 1984. $1.45.
_____. "Serum Lipids, Prostaglandins, and Marine Oils." *J.
    of the International Academy of Preventive Medicine* 3
    (1983): 16–22.
Breslow, L., and N. Belloc. "Relationship of Physical Health
    Status and Health Practices." *Preventive Medicine* 1
    (1972): 409–21.
Bull, R. "Low Calcium, Chlorine, and Fat Linked to Heart
    Disease." *Science News* 124 (1983): 103.
Burkitt, D., A. Walker, and N. Painter. "Effects of Dietary
    Fiber on Stool and Transit Times, and Its Role in the
    Causation of Disease." *Lancet* 10 (1972): 1408–11.
Carlson, A. H. and F. Hoelzel. "Apparent Prolongation of the
    Life Span of Rats by Intermittent Fasting." *J. Nutrition*
    31 (1946): 363.
Carpenter, D., and J. Hart. "Toward an Integrated Theory of
    Aging." *American Laboratory* (April 1971): 48–52.
Chen, W. L., and J. W. Anderson. "Effects of Plant Fiber in
    Decreasing Plasma Total Cholesterol and Increasing
    High-Density Lipoprotein Cholesterol." *Proc. Soc. Exp.
    Biol. Med.* 162 (1979): 310–14.
Cheney, K. E., R. U. Lie, G. S. Smith, R. E. Leung, N. R.
    Nickey, and R. L. Walford. "Survival and Disease Pat-
    terns in C57B1/6J Mice Subject to Undernutrition." *Exp.
    Gerontol.* 15 (1980): 237–39.
Cheraskin, E. "Influence of Nutrients on Behavior." Paper
    read at the Meeting of the International Academy of
    Preventive Medicine (1975) at Los Angeles.
Cheraskin, E. and W. M. Ringsdorf. "Homeostasis: The Crux

of the Prevention Problem." *J. of the International Academy of Preventive Medicine* 2 (July 1982): 25–52.

Cheraskin, E., W. M. Ringsdorf, and A. Brecher. *Psychodietetics.* New York: Stein and Day, 1974.

Cheraskin, E., W. Ringsdorf, and F. Medford. "The Ideal Daily Vitamin A Intake." *Int. J. Vitamin Nutr. Research* 1 (1976): 58–60.

Clar, E. J. and A. Fourtanier. "L'acide Pyrrolidone Carboxylique (PCA) et la Peau." *Int. J. Cosmetic Science* 3 (1981): 101–13.

Clayman, C. and D. O'Reilly. "Jejunoileal Bypass: Pass It By." *JAMA* 9 (August 28, 1981): 988.

Coker, Charles. "Cytotoxic Testing." *Information Bulletin of the Health and Tennis Corporation of America,* Dr. Paul Ward, editor (1983): 1 and 6.

Columbu, Drs. Anita and Franco. *Redesign Your Body: The 90-Day Real Body Makeover.* New York: E. P. Dutton, 1984.

Colvin, R. H. and S. B. Olson. "A Descriptive Analysis of Men and Women Who Have Lost Significant Weight and Are Highly Successful at Maintaining the Loss." *Addict. Behav.* 3 (1983): 287–95.

Cureton, T. "Nutritive Aspects of Physical Fitness Work." *Swimming Technique* 6 (1969): 44–49.

————. "Wheat Germ Oil, the 'Wonder' Fuel." *Scholastic Coach* 24 (March 1955): 36.

DeLuise, M., G. Blackburn, and J. Flier. "Reduced Activity of the Red-cell Sodium Potassium Pump in Human Obesity." *New Eng. J. of Med.* 19 (October 1980): 1017–22.

Edelstein, B. *The Woman Doctor's Diet for Women.* New York: Prentice Hall, 1977.

Fairburn, C. (Warneford Hospital, Oxford, England). "A Cognitive Behavioral Approach to the Treatment of Bulimia." *Psychological Medicine* 4 (November 1981): 707–11.

Faserberg, B., O. Andersson, U. Nilsson, T. Hedner, B. Isaksson, and P. Bjerntorp. "Weight-reducing Diets: Role of Carbohydrates on Sympathetic Nervous Activity and Hypotensive Response." *Int. J. Obes.* 3 (1984): 237–43.

Finch, E. E. and L. Hayflick, editors. *The Handbook of the Biology of Aging.* New York: Van Nostrand Reinhold, 1977: 159.

Fujimoto, D. "Aging and Cross-linking in Human Aorta." *Biochemical and Biophysical Research Communications* 4 (December 1982): 1264–69.

Gallup Youth Survey. "Third of Teens Skip Breakfast." *Los Angeles Times* report, II (November 9, 1977): 5.

Graeber, C., J. Goust, A. Glassman, R. Kendall, and C. Loadholt. "Immunomodulating Properties of Dimethylglycine in Humans." *J. of Infectious Diseases* 1 (January 1981): 101–5.

Grant, E. "Food Allergy and Migraine." *Lancet* (May 1979): 966–68.

Greist, J. "Exercise in the Prevention and Treatment of Depression." Paper presented at the meeting of the American College of Sports Medicine (1980), Wash. D.C.

Hager, D. "Implanatation von Fetalem Thymusgewebe zur Steigerung der Koerpersigenen Abwehr." *Cytobiological Review* 3 (1984): 144–50.

Hartman, D. "The Free Radical Theory of Aging." *J. Geront.* 12 (1957): 257–59.

Harper, Harold. *How You Can Beat the Killer Diseases.* Westport, CT: Arlington House, 1977.

Hofeldt, F. and E. Lufkin. "Are Abnormalities in Insulin Secretion Responsible for Reactive Hypoglycemia?" *Diabetes* vol. 23, no. 7 (1974): 589–95.

Holistic and Preventive UP-DATE, newsletter published by the International Academy of Holistic Health and Medicine. 218 Avenue B, Redondo Beach, CA 90277.

Horrobin, D. F., M. S. Manku, M. Oka, R. O. Morgan, S. C. Cunnane, A. I. Ally, T. Ghayur, M. Schweitzer, and R. A. Karmali. "The Nutritional Regulation of T Lymphocyte Function." *Medical Hypothesis* 5 (1979): 969–85.

Horton, E. S. "Metabolic Aspects of Exercise and Weight Reduction." 31st Annual Meeting of the American College of Sports Medicine (May 1984), San Diego, California.

Horvath, P. and C. Ip. "Synergistic Effect of Vitamin E and

Selenium in the Chemoprevention of Mammary Carcinogenesis in Rats." *Cancer Research* 43 (1983): 5335–41.

Hudiburgh, N. K. "A Multidisciplinary Approach to Weight Control." *J. Am. Diet. Assoc.* 4 (1984): 447–50.

Hylander, B. and S. Rossner. "Effects of Dietary Fiber Intake Before Meals on Weight Loss and Hunger in a Weight-reducing Club." *Acta Med. Scand.* 3 (1983): 217–20.

Jeffery, R. W., W. M. Bjornson-Benson, B. S. Rosenthal, R. A. Lindquist, C. L. Kurth, and S. L. Johnson. "Correlates of Weight Loss and Its Maintenance Over Two Years of Follow-up Among Middle-aged men." *Prev. Med.* 2 (March 1984): 155–68.

Katch, F., W. McArdle, and B. Boylan. *Getting in Shape*. Boston: Houghton Mifflin, 1979.

Kramsch, D. M., A. Aspen, and L. Rozler; "Atherosclerosis: Prevention by Agents Not Affecting Abnormal Levels of Blood Lipids." *Science* 213 (1981): 1511–14.

Kugler, H. "Are You a Victim of Bulimia?" Survey questionnaire published in the *Health Express* (August 1983).

———. "The Combination Theory of Aging." *American Laboratory* (April 1978): 38–44.

———. "Diet and Health Habits as Related to the Onset of Disease." *J. IAPM* (Winter 1977): 68–76.

———. *Dr. Kugler's Seven Keys to a Longer Life*. New York: Stein and Day, 1978.

———. "Food Frequency Intake, Exercise, and Muscle Mass in Bulimics." Paper in preparation.

———. "The Importance of Exercise in the Treatment of Bulimia." Research performed at the Health Integration Center, Torrance, California. Paper in preparation.

———. *The Weight and Appetite Control Workbook*. Redondo Beach, CA: International Academy of Holistic Health and Medicine, 1985.

Lamb, L. "Muscle Loss from Weight Loss." *The Health Letter* 5 (1977): 1–2.

Lampman, R. "Exercise as a Partial Therapy for the Grossly Obese." 31st annual meeting of the American College of Sports Medicine (May 1984), San Diego, California.

Lansing, A. I., editor. *Cowdry's Problems of Ageing*, 3rd ed. New York: William and William, 1952: 139.

Lukaski, H. C. "Assessment of Fat-Free Mass Using Bioelectrical Impedance Measurements of the Human Body." *Am. J. Clinical Nutrition* 39 (1984): 658–63.

Marston, J. "Effects of Excessive Caloric Intake and Caloric Restriction on Body Weight and Energy Expenditure at Rest and Light Exercise." *Acta Physiol. Scand.* 114 (January 1982): 2043–55.

Merimee, E. "Arginine-initiated Release of Human Growth Hormone." *New Engl. J. Med.* 280 (1969): 1434–38.

Middleton, J. D. and M. F. Roberts. "Effect of a Skin Cream Containing the Sodium Salts of Pyrrolidone Carboxylic Acid on Dry and Flaky Skin." *J. Soc. Cosmet. Chem.* 29 (1978): 201–5.

Mitchell, J. E., R. Pyle, and D. Elke. "Frequency and Duration of Binge-eating Episodes in Patients with Bulimia." *Amer. J. Psychiatry* 6 (June 1981): 835–36.

Mooney, P. *The Supernutrition Handbook.* Supernutrition Research, 531-44th Avenue, San Francisco, CA 94121. $6.00.

J. Morris, S. Chase, C. Adam, C. Sirey, B. Tech, L. Epstein, and D. Sheehan. "Vigorous Exercise in Leisure-time and the Incidence of Coronary Heart Disease." *Lancet* 1 (1973): 333–38.

Ornish, D. "Good Health Practices: An Effective Means in Preventing Heart Disease." *JAMA* (January 7, 1983): 54.

Oscai, L. B. "Exercise and Weight Reduction in the Obese Rat." 31st annual meeting of the American College of Sports Medicine (May 1984), San Diego, California.

Packer, L. and J. Smith. "Extension of the In-Vitro Lifespan of Human WI-38 Cells by Vitamin E." Paper read at the 4th Annual Meeting of the American Aging Association (1974), Los Angeles, California.

Pascher, G. "Die Wasserloeslichen Bestandteile der Peripheren Hornschicht (Hautoberflaeche) Quantitative Analysen, Pyrrolidoncarbonsaeure." *Arch. Klin. Exp. Dermatol.* 203 (1956): 234–38.

Passwater, R. *The Easy No-Flab Diet*. New York: Marek, 1979.

———. *Selenium as Food and Medicine*. New Canaan: Keats Publishing, 1981.

———. *Supernutrition for Healthy Hearts*. New York: Dial Press, 1977.

Passwater, R. and E. Cranton. *Trace Elements, Hair Analysis and Nutrition*. New Canaan: Keats Publishing, 1983.

Pearl, R. *The Rate of Living Theory of Aging*. New York: Knopf, 1928.

Picot, D., D. Rolland, and R. Hellegouarch. "Lean Body Mass and Body Fat Evaluation by Electrical Impedancemetry." *Medica Jadertina (Jugoslavia)*, VIth Int. Conf. on Electrical Bio-Impedance (September 1983), Belgrade.

Pyle, R. L., J. E. Mitchell, and E. Eckert. "Bulimia: A Report of 34 Cases." *J. Clin. Psychiatry* 2 (February 1981): 60–64.

Reinhardt, J. "Biochemical Pathology Initiated by Free Radicals, Oxidant Chemicals, and Therapeutic Drugs in the Etiology of Chemical Hypersensitivity Disease." *J. Orthomolecular Psychiat*. 12 (1983): 166–83.

Reuben, D. *The Save Your Life Diet*. New York: Random House, 1976.

Rodale, R. "Polluted Rats Turn to Drink." *Rodale's Health Bulletin* 8 (July 25, 1970): 2.

Rosch, P. "Stress and Cardiovascular Disease." *Comprehensive Therapy* 9 (1983): 6–13.

Rucker, R. D., E. K. Chan, J. Horstmann, E. P. Chute, R. L. Varco, and H. Buchwald. "Searching for the Best Weight Reduction Operation." *Surgery* 4 (October 1984): 624–31.

Russ, C. S., P. A. Ciavarella, and R. L. Atkinson. "A Comprehensive Outpatient Weight Reduction Program: Dietary Patterns, Psychological considerations, and Treatment Principles." *J. Am. Diet. Assoc*. 4 (April 1984): 444–46.

Schnare, D. "Body Burden Reduction of PCBs, PBBs and Chlorinated Pesticides in Human Subjects." *Ambio* 13 (1983): 378–80.

Schrauzer, G. N., J. E. McGinness, and K. Kuehn. "Effects of

Selenium Supplementation on the Genesis of Spontaneous Mammary Tumors in Inbred C3H/St Mice." *Carcinogenesis* (London) 1 (1980): 199–201.

Scrimshaw, N. "An Analysis of Past and Present Recommended Dietary Allowances for Protein in Health and Disease." *New Eng. J. Med.* 4 (1976): 198–203.

Selye, H. "Stress, Cancer, and Behavior." *J. Int. Academy of Preventive Medicine* 1 (1982): 17–23.

_____. *Stress Without Distress.* New York: Signet Books, 1975.

_____. "Stress and Aging." *J. of the Amer. Geriatr. Soc.* 18 (1970): 669–80.

Scheldahl, L. "Special Ergometric Techniques and Weight Reduction." 31st annual meeting of the American College of Sports Medicine (May 1984), San Diego, California.

Smythies, J. "The Biochemistry of Psychosis." *Scottish Medical J.* vol. 15, no. 1 (1970): 34–37.

Stern, J. S. "Useful Animal Models and Techniques in the Study of Exercise and Obesity." 31st annual meeting of the American College of Sports Medicine (May 1984), San Diego, California. Still, J. "A Cybernetic Theory of Aging." *Med. Ann. Dstr Columbia* 25 (1964): 199.

Strehler, B. "Aging: Transcriptional and Translational Control Mechanisms and Their Alteration." Paper read at the 140th Meeting of the American Association for the Advancement of Science (1974), San Francisco, California.

Sussman, K. "Plasma Insulin Levels During Reactive Hypoglycemia." *Diabetes* vol. 15, no. 1 (1966): 1–4.

Wald, N. J., J. Boreham, J. L. Hayward, and R. D. Bulbrook. "Plasma Retinol, Beta-carotene and Vitamin E Levels in Relation to the Future Risk of Breast Cancer." *Br. J. Cancer* 49 (1984): 321–24.

Wald, N. J., M. Idle, and J. Boreham. "Low Serum Vitamin A and Subsequent Risk of Cancer." *Lancet* 2 (1980): 813–15.

Walford, R. "The Immunologic Theory of Aging." *Gerontologist* 4 (1964): 195–201.

_____. *Maximum Life Span.* New York: W. W. Norton, 1984.

Ward, J. *Emotional Aspects of Hypoglycemia in Endocrinology and Diabetes.* New York: Grune and Stratton, 1975.

Webb, P. "Direct Calorimetry and the Energetics of Exercise and Weight Reduction." Annual meeting of the American College of Sports Medicine (May 1984), San Diego, California.

Weindruch, R. H., S. R. Gottesman, and R. L. Walford. "Modification of Age-related Immune Decline in Mice Dietarily Restricted from or after Mid-adulthood." *Proc. Nat. Acad. Sci. U.S.A.* 79 (1982): 898–99.

Weinsier, R. L., T. A. Wadden, C. Ritenbaugh, G. Harrison, F. S. Johnson, and J. H. Wilmore, "Recommended therapeutic Guidelines for Professional Weight Control Programs." *Am. J. Clin. Nutr.* 4 (1984): 865–72.

Yaryura, J. A. and F. A. Neziroglu. "Psychosis and Disturbance of Glucose Metabolism." Paper presented at the meeting of the Society of Biological Psychiatry (June 6, 1974), Boston, Massachusetts.

Index